SF 0 9 '09

P9-DEB-045

Allergy and Celiac Diets

With

EASE

616.9750654
DUM

Money and Time Saving Solutions for Food Allergy and Gluten-Free Diets

Nicolette M. Dumke

BARRINGTON AREA LIBRARY
505 N. NORTHWEST HWY.
BARRINGTON, ILLINOIS 60010

ALLERG   **SE, REVISED**
MONE   **TIONS**
FOR FOOD ALLERGY AND GLUTEN-FREE DIETS

All rights reserved. No part of this book may be reproduced or transmitted in any form or by any means, electronic or mechanical, including photocopying, recording, or by any information storage and retrieval system without written permission from the author, except for the inclusion of brief quotations in a review.

Published by
Adapt Books
Allergy Adapt, Inc.
1877 Polk Avenue
Louisville, Colorado 80027
303-666-8253

©2009 by Nicolette M. Dumke
First edition ©2008
Printed in the United States of America

Publisher's Cataloging-in-Publication
(Provided by Quality Books, Inc.)

Dumke, Nicolette M.
   Allergy and celiac diets with ease : money and time saving solutions for food allergy and gluten-free diets / Nicolette M. Dumke.
   238 p. 24.4 cm.
   Includes bibliographical references and index.
   LCCN 2008911641
   ISBN-13: 978-1-887624-17-6
   ISBN-10: 1-887624-17-1

   1. Food allergy--Diet therapy--Recipes. 2. Celiac disease--Diet therapy--Recipes. I. Title.

RC588.D53D85 2008   641.5'6318
                QBI07-600278

Dedication

To Mark, Joel, and John

Thank you for all the joy
you bring into my life.

Disclaimer

The information contained in this book is merely intended to communicate food preparation material and information about possible treatment options which are helpful and educational to the reader. It is not intended to replace medical diagnosis or treatment, but rather to provide information and recipes which may be helpful in implementing a diet prescribed by your doctor. Please consult your physician for medical advice before embarking on any treatment or changing your diet.

The author and publisher declare that to the best of their knowledge all material in this book is accurate; however, although unknown to the author and publisher, some recipes may contain ingredients which may be harmful to some people.

There are no warranties which extend beyond the educational nature of this book, either expressed or implied, including, but not limited to, the implied warranties of merchantability, fitness for a particular purpose, or non-infringement. Therefore, the author and publisher shall have neither liability nor responsibility to any person with respect to any loss or damage alleged to be caused, directly or indirectly, by the information contained in this book.

If you do not wish to be bound by the above, you may return this book to the publisher for a full refund.

Table of Contents

Foreword

When you pick up this book, you really are getting two books: one of information about food allergy and celiac diets and how to live on them without breaking the bank and also a book of recipes that you can use on your diet. In the first book you can benefit from Nickie's vast experience to quickly gain information that it would take years to gather on your own. This part of the book provides an understanding of food allergies and celiac disease, the importance of your special diet and of food safety to long-term health, and information about economizing, shopping, organizing, and cooking with ease.

The second part of the book is recipes tailored to make your meals tasty while also loaded with nutrition. Aware of the time and financial pressures of busy modern lives, Nickie has streamlined all recipes to make cooking easier. The reference sections offer added information about where to find gluten-free and allergen-free foods. The many easy recipes in this book should go far to reducing the stress of a difficult diet.

Anyone can learn from the ideas presented. Do you need motivation to tackle and implement a food allergy or celiac diet? Be sure to read the section, "The How and Why of Your Diet." This section, as well as the reference section on food safety, can make dining out a safer and more healthy experience. The "Time-Saving Solutions" chapter gives information that will help those with celiac disease or food allergies find a restaurant that can prepare the gluten-free or allergen-free food they need and have a pleasant dining-out experience without a reaction. The "Cooking With Ease" and "Baking With Ease" chapters tell how to get organized for cooking and baking and do it with the least amount of time and effort. These chapters are loaded with gems of information from Nickie's more than thirty years of experience in cooking for special diets.

All of us would be healthier and more energetic if we incorporated some of the alternative foods this book presents such as nutritious non-grains and non-sugar sweeteners into our diets. Put this book to good use and you will find not only that your health will improve but that you are also saving money and time on preparing your meals. You will enjoy your meals – and life – more.

Ann Fisk, B.S., R.N.
Founder of *An Ounce of Prevention*

Introduction to the Revised Edition

The original *Allergy and Celiac Diets With Ease* is about a year old at the time of this writing. I never expected to revise a book this soon because I normally lack enough new information for a revision to be important in less than several years.

The information available for this book has not changed much in the last year, but the circumstances we Americans find ourselves in have changed dramatically. Our financial crisis has deepened into a recession with the dreaded "D" word on everyone's mind across the globe. As I have watched the changes and listened to people's reactions to them, I realized that I'm old enough to know some things that keep me from being adversely affected by the changes as much as many younger people are.

Because my parents grew up during the Great Depression, I, as a child, was immersed in Great-Depression-born habits and ways of doing things. I have retained many of these habits and applied them to all areas of my life, including my special diet. These 75-year old ideas are "up to the minute" and exactly what we need now. I had them a year ago when I finished the first version of this book, but I did not include most of them because I did not realize readers would need them in the near future. Since these ideas are relevant now, this revision was written to share the wisdom of my forbears.

What's to Eat?

"What's for dinner?" This perennial question becomes more difficult to answer when you or a family member must follow a diet that eliminates wheat, gluten, milk, yeast, corn, soy or other foods that are the basic ingredients of standard fare. When you combine the demands of a special diet with financial pressure and the hurried pace of modern life, making dinner (or breakfast, or lunch, or muffins that "fit" your diet) may seem nearly impossible at times.

This book will help you cook for your special diet as economically, quickly, and easily as possible but in ways different from other sources you may have consulted. If you look in other cookbooks for quick ways to make a meal, the advice you may find can sound like this:

> A can of this,
> A can of that,
> A can of mushroom soup,
> Some biscuit mix,
> Some processed cheese,
> And there's your dinner, made with ease!

Can this really be a recipe for dinner or is it a recipe for fake food? Even though it is made at home, the component ingredients are so highly processed that you don't get optimal nutrition. And of course this food usually does not conform to an allergy or celiac diet; a recipe like this is a serious threat to health for some of us. Real food is good for everyone's health (even those who are not on special diets), tastes better, and is more economical. We just need to know how to cook it in limited time and purchase the ingredients we need with limited money.

So how can we economize and stay on our special diets without spending all day in the kitchen? First, accept the fact that you *will* be doing some cooking. Learn to enjoy the creativity of it rather than regretting the time spent. Then organize and simplify. Use money and time-saving practices, appliances, gadgets, and wholesome ingredients. (This book will introduce you to these helpers). Finally, use the right recipes. This book contains recipes for simple, wholesome foods, simply but flavorfully prepared. Skip recipes with dozens of ingredients. Skip the cream of mushroom soup and other highly processed foods. As you follow this book, you will find yourself saving money and enjoying simple wholesome foods while you enjoy improved health.

The How and Why of Your Diet

People who have been recently diagnosed with food allergies or celiac disease respond to the news of their condition in a number of ways. The most common reaction I hear is that of being overwhelmed by the complexity of the diet they are supposed to follow and the changes it will make in every day life. They ask the question, "*How* do I do this?" (This question will be answered in the next several chapters). Another reaction is relief that a cause for their poor health has been found and that the prognosis is not serious as long as they stay on the diet.

Some patients also ask, "*Why* do I have to be on this diet?" Learning the answer to this question will help motivate you to be diligent about staying on your diet and will get you going when it is time to cook. For both celiacs and those with food allergies, the most convincing way for you to answer this question for yourself is to stay on your diet diligently for a few weeks or months and see how you feel. The improved health you are likely to experience – sometimes after just a few days on the diet – is the most basic and important reason, and one that even children understand and find motivating.

Celiac disease is more well defined than food allergies, both in the diagnosis and understanding of the illness and in the uniformity of the diet. The medical definition of celiac disease is a genetic condition in which the patient has antibodies to gluten. These antibodies cause an immune response in the intestine when gluten is eaten, which results in damage to the intestinal villi. This damage leads to maldigestion, intestinal distress, and malabsorption of nutrients. Although blood tests are used to detect the presence of antibodies to the components of gluten, the first part of the gold standard test for celiac disease is having an intestinal biopsy which shows the characteristic damage to the intestine.

The malabsorption of nutrients caused by celiac disease can lead to other problems such as anemia, osteoporosis, fatigue, weakness, muscle cramps, neurological symptoms, and even some forms of cancer. (This list is included here because it will motivate you to stay on your diet!) The only treatment is lifelong strict avoidance of gluten. After the patient has avoided gluten for several months, the intestine heals and the effects of the disease are reversed. The reversal of symptoms is the second part of the gold standard criteria for the diagnosis of celiac disease. If improvement does not occur or is not complete, the possibility of intolerance to other foods such as milk may be considered.

The celiac diet is "simple" to the doctor who tells you to follow it – just avoid gluten. The more helpful doctor will elaborate by telling you to avoid wheat, rye, barley, and possibly oats. While not simple in practice, at least the celiac diet is easily defined. This makes it possible for health food producers and supplement manufacturers to make products for the gluten-intolerant. The August 2007 issue of *Better Nutrition* reported that more than 2500 gluten-free products line the shelves of health food stores. Restaurants which cater to the gluten-intolerant are springing up in large cities as more and more people are being diagnosed with gluten intolerance. If a person with celiac disease has enough money to regularly purchase commercially prepared gluten-free foods (which is unlikely in these tough economic times), does not have or develop any other intolerances (such as to rice, the basic ingredient of most gluten-free food), and lives in a city large enough to support gluten-free restaurants, life can go on as before diagnosis with some relatively minor changes and modification. However, if your budget is restricted or you live in a small town, you will need to learn new ways of cooking and eating.

Food allergies pose a different situation. They are a poor cousin to celiac disease in terms of respect from the conventional medical community. In my opinion, this is because food allergy is a diverse problem which usually does not have a well-defined or easy solution. The immunological mediators of food allergies (often called sensitivities if they do not involve IgE antibodies) are diverse, the foods a person is likely to be intolerant of can be a long, complex list, and the conditions that may caused by food allergies are many. Average doctors (who practice as though "for every ill there is a pill") find this overwhelming so they often make light of food allergies. However, food allergies are just as real as celiac disease, and they also can result in malnutrition, anemia, osteoporosis, and other serious conditions. For more about the definition, diagnosis, treatment, and conditions that can be associated with food allergies, see *The Ultimate Food Allergy Cookbook and Survival Guide* as described on the last pages of this book.

Another question people recently diagnosed with food allergies often ask themselves is, "Why am I doing all this cooking?" Even if they can afford to purchase commercially prepared foods routinely, people with multiple food allergies usually must be able to do some cooking for themselves because there are not enough people with the same combination of food allergies to support a special segment of the health food industry as there is for celiacs. The more foods allergy patients are allergic to and the more complex their diets are, the more they will be unable to rely on commercial food producers and restaurants for their meals. Celiacs who do not want to spend over $6 for a small loaf of bread also will benefit from cooking for themselves. In addition, some celiacs develop intolerance to rice, milk, or other foods. In these cases, they are faced with the same challenges as people with multiple food allergies. Finally, the wisest celiacs learn from the experiences of others and cook for themselves instead of relying solely on commercially prepared foods so that they can eat a variety of grains and grain alternatives rather than eating rice-containing foods at every meal. Thus, they lessen their chances of developing sensitivity to rice and probably will be able to preserve their ability to eat out occasionally and eat commercially prepared foods when they are temporarily too busy to cook.

The best reason to cook for yourself is because that is the only way to have real control of your diet. As the restaurant dining tip sheet of the Gluten Intolerance Group of North America says, "The only person who really knows what went into a dish is the person who made it!" If you are the cook, and you are starting with known ingredients, then and only then can you know that you are totally safe.

Although the next chapter offers information on how to eat in a restaurant, it never possible to be 100% certain that you are really getting what you asked for. I have had reactions after eating only *plain* buffalo and a *plain uncut* baked potato in a restaurant. This means that something was not plain! Most restaurants cater to normal customers and are staffed by healthy people who taste what they serve and possibly cannot believe that anyone would want meat as dry as some buffalo. I suspect that they shop around until they find "buffalo" that is more tender, and that they thus inadvertently purchase meat which has been larded with beef or pork fat. Or perhaps it is marinated or otherwise chemically tenderized without the knowledge of the staff member who assures you that it is plain.

In addition, if you find a restaurant that is special-diet-aware, you cannot relax your diligence. You must remind them every time of exactly what you need. A restaurant that is good today may not be good tomorrow. Staff turnover may occur, and the restaurant is only as good as its weakest employee.

A final important reason for everyone – even the healthy and wealthy – to cook for themselves most of the time is the prevention of illness. Usually the food borne illnesses acquired in restaurants are mild. However, some of the most allergic people I talk to developed food allergies after a bout with a parasitic disease. These people are often allergic to chemicals as well as foods, must live in isolation, and have little hope of ever recovering even partially. With global travel and immigration, you do not have to visit a Third World country to contract a parasite. The world and its parasites will come to you.

It is estimated that 80% of people with food allergies suffer from some degree of impairment of hydrochloric acid secretion by their stomach.* In addition to its role in the digestion of food, hydrochloric acid serves to nearly sterilize food before it enters the small intestine. Therefore, due to no or an inadequate level of hydrochloric acid, most people with food allergies have much less defense against parasites and other food borne illnesses than a healthy person.

*Braly, James, M.D. *Dr. Braly's Food Allergy and Nutrition Revolution.* Keats Publishing, New Haven, CT, 1992, page 73.

I do not eat anything in a restaurant that is not cooked just before serving and served piping hot because my food allergies were probably triggered by a parasitic infection. I never left the country, but I did eat in restaurants where I had no control over the hand-washing habits of the employees, some of whom were undoubtedly from parts of the world where the parasite I contracted is endemic and is carried by almost every member of the population without major ill effects.

Restaurant employees are not the only possible contributors to food borne infections. If you eat at a salad bar, you have no control over what other diners might have put into the salad fixings before you got there. Recent scares with *E. coli* on pre-washed table-ready fresh vegetables implicated a very reputable organic farming corporation. You cannot be too safe with your food. At our house produce which will be eaten raw is decontaminated by soaking in a sink full of water plus Nutribiotic™ (See "Sources," page 209). For more on eating out safely see the next chapter of this book. For more about safe food handling practices at home, see pages 215 to 218.

In addition to microbial food safety, ingredient control, and strict kitchen food separation habits to eliminate gluten or allergen contamination of foods, there are other food health issues which are beyond the scope of this book. They include pesticides on food and genetically engineering of foods which may introduce a gene from a food to which you are allergic into a food that appears to be one of your safe foods. (For more information about this, see *Chemical-Free Kids: The Organic Sequel* which is listed in "References," page 221). The best way to control exposure to these factors is to shop carefully and cook for yourself most of the time.

Eating out when you are on a special diet is like flying. If what you eat is likely to be safe from infectious organisms (i.e. freshly prepared, thoroughly cooked, and served piping hot), you have celiac disease but no other intolerances, and you are eating at a restaurant awarded three stars by the Gluten-Free Restaurant Awareness Program (described in the next chapter) at a less-busy time of day, it is like flying in a commercial aircraft – likely to be safe. If you have multiple food allergies or eat unsafe foods, eating out can be like flying a glider near the Rocky Mountains where there are unpredictable updrafts. Although it is fun and relaxing to eat out occasionally if your diet and budget allow, it is best for your health to cook at home most of the time. The less often you fly (or eat out), the less likely you are to crash (have a reaction or contract a food borne illness). Cooking for yourself routinely is not as difficult or time consuming as you may think. The rest of this book will show you how to do it more easily.

Money-Saving Solutions

Food is a basic necessity of life, and how nutritiously we eat profoundly influences our health. When money is tight, we cannot quit eating. The question is how to spend money on food wisely and receive an adequate quantity of food with the best nutritional value for our budget. Nutritionists often talk about nutrient-dense food, meaning food that contains the most nutrients for the number of calories. If we adapt that idea and think about maximizing nutrients per dollar, it will put how we spend our food money into the proper perspective.

At the time of this writing, American has just officially moved into a recession which we hope will not become a depression. It is my fervent hope and prayer that every reader of this book has sufficient income, reserve in a bank account, or access to a government or charitable safety net to make it possible for her or him to eat well and feed a family healthily. This chapter will help you to carefully and efficiently use your money for food and hopefully prevent the need for literally tightening your belt due to less-than-adequate nutrition.

Guard Your Health

The most important way to save money is to be healthy. For those of us with food allergies or gluten intolerance, eating economically cannot mean eating less expensive foods that do not fit our special diets. If you are gluten-intolerant, cheating on your diet can damage your intestine and eventually lead to serious health consequences. As discussed in the last chapter, because celiac disease is a well-defined condition, there is data correlating this disease with other conditions. Thus, medical experts know with certainty that uncontrolled celiac disease (i.e. when the diet is not followed diligently) can lead to malnutrition, osteoporosis, anemia, neurological conditions, and even some forms of cancer. Food allergies can also damage the intestinal lining causing some of the consequences above to occur. If you develop serious medical problems, even if you are insured, you will spend much more on medical bills than you might save on food if you eat foods which you do not tolerate. In addition, if you are not healthy, you will find it harder to function, do your work well, or enjoy friends and family.

Everyone's health, even that of seemingly healthy people, is influenced by what they eat. Diets that are high in sugar and unhealthy fats can lead to obesity, heart disease, diabetes, and other serious conditions. If the food you eat contains infectious organisms, you may get bacterial food poisoning (usually short-lived and not serious unless caused by enteropathogenic *E. coli*), contract a viral illness (which may either be transient or lead to long-term problems), or pick up a parasite which can lead to long-lasting consequences such as food allergies and chemical sensitivities. To be sure your food is safe to eat, all animal foods must be thoroughly cooked. If you have insufficient hydrochloric acid production in your stomach, as do many people with food allergies, plant foods should also be cooked or disinfected before eating them raw. See pages 217 for more about how to disinfect produce and about food safety in general.

When you cook for yourself, YOU are in control of everything you eat. You can choose foods that have the highest nutrient density per dollar, make certain that the fats and sweeteners you use are healthy and used in reasonable amounts, and use good food safety practices to insure that your food is safe. This is the best way to safeguard your health.

Set Up a Budget

My parents grew up during the Great Depression which forced them to develop frugal habits. When I got my first job after college, my mother gave me a spiral notebook and a lesson on how to keep track of how and where I was spending my money and then use that information to set up a budget. My husband's family did not use a budget, so when we were first married and were DINKs (**D**ouble **I**ncome, although his income was a graduate student's stipend, with **No Ki**ds), we did not have a budget. However, I did cook everything from scratch and taught my husband more nutritious eating habits rooted in my agricultural Italian heritage. We owned one car and lived close enough to my husband's school that he could walk or ride a bike to get there. (This was good exercise as well as a way to save money). We lived in a small apartment and saved diligently for a house.

When we had our children, we were living on my husband's income only. I was impressed with the need to plan ahead for their college education, so I went back to the old notebook budget system with a certain amount of money allocated from every paycheck for each category of expenses. Returning to budgeting was an eye-opener for me. I was amazed at how much I had spent on gifts for people I was not even especially close to (such as baby gifts for former co-workers). We had a few other "great realizations" about where money was going as well. These realizations caused us to close the loopholes, and we tweaked our budget for a few months until it fit our actual expenses and needs. We have lived on a budget ever since. Naturally, money allocations in our budget needed occasional adjustment, but the only change we have made in how we manage our budget over the years is to replace the spiral notebooks with Excel files on the computer which make the time spent managing the budget briefer and the arithmetic easier.

Although using a budget can seem constraining if you have never done it before, it is actually extremely liberating in the long run. It makes you aware of where your money is going and you can use that information to make wise decisions. For example, because we knew exactly how much we spent on gas, we chose to drive small fuel-efficient cars. When the price of gasoline began to skyrocket, we were in much better shape than our neighbors who owned SUVs and vans. After you have been on a budget and made decisions based on what you have learned from it for a number of years, you may find yourself free of debt (except possibly a mortgage) and able to buy large items like cars with cash, thus saving an incredible amount of money on interest. Such purchasing is truly liberating.

My younger son recently reminded me of something about his childhood. Both of our sons received a modest allowance every week. We had them donate a small amount, and they could spend the rest on whatever they wanted. When we went to Target once a week, they usually spent their allowances on toys. As they grew older, they wanted larger toys that cost more money than they had that week. My son recently reminded me that, although he often begged me, I never gave him extra money or even an advance on his allowance to buy a more expensive toy. He had to save up his allowance until he had enough to buy the toy he wanted. As our sons reached their late elementary school years, we witnessed some several-month saving sprees for large space Lego™ sets. Children (at least sons – I have no experience with daughters) raised this way actually prefer non-designer clothing, and our sons voluntarily included economics in the factors they considered when they chose colleges. Between their wise choices and the saving programs we began for them at birth, they will both graduate from college debt-free. Currently, they save about 90% of their pay from summer jobs and have bought cars using cash. My only financial concern about our sons is whether they will be able find wives who can adjust to their frugality!

The "moral" of this story about our family is that although the current financial crisis is hard for many Americans, if it forces us to return to the frugal habits of our parents or grandparents and teach them to our children, the long-term result may be positive. Americans have become conspicuous consumers over the last few decades, but possessions do not bring us true happiness. A re-ordering of priorities may be what is needed for many reasons beyond just allowing us to survive the recession.

Here are a few practical considerations for budgeting: Be realistic when you plan a budget, yet try to be frugal. Expect to have to adjust your budget for the first several months to make it fit your actual expenses rather than your ideas of how much you are spending in each category. You will also have to adjust your budget whenever there is a change in your circumstances or new priorities arise. Set aside a little money from each paycheck for unexpected expenses or emergencies.

In your grocery budget, allow enough money to buy sufficient nutritious food because good nutrition is the basis of good health. If what you have to spend does not cover everything you would normally buy, skip foods that provide mostly empty calories such as some snacks and beverages. Make homemade soda pop for your children by mixing carbonated water with fruit juice concentrate. (See the recipe on page 174). This refreshing beverage provides sound nutritional value as well as saving money.

As you begin to track expenditures with a budget, the cumulative expense of a daily stop at Starbucks™ or a similar coffee shop on the way to work may shock you. To save money make your own coffee at home and put it in a insulated travel mug to take to work. There are many good automatic coffee makers on the market, some of which come in small or single-serving sizes. You can set up the coffee maker in the evening, plug it in the next morning, and have your coffee made in a few minutes with very little effort. If you do not have an automatic coffee maker, an inexpensive French drip system also makes delicious coffee. See the coffee recipe on page 173 for more about this method of making coffee.

If you must save time in addition to money, consider using instant coffee. Mount Hagen organic instant coffee is delicious and rich-tasting yet costs only $7.75 for a 60-serving bottle at the time of this writing. Even if you take a large mug with a double-sized serving of coffee, cream, and sweetener, your coffee will cost less than 50 cents per day and, without a stop at the coffee shop, you will save time in the morning as well.

Snacks and beverages are an area of the grocery budget where we often receive the lowest nutrient density per dollar, so consider making these foods at home. See pages 173 to 181 for recipes for economical homemade snacks and beverages.

Have a Plan When You Grocery Shop

An almost certain way to have more month than grocery money is to routinely walk into the grocery store at the end of the day without a plan. To save money, you must be organized and plan ahead. Never go to the grocery store when you are hungry. If you cannot go right after a meal, at least have a snack before you enter the store. If you are hungry, you will tempted to buy the high priced goodies which are so attractively displayed in prominent places. Buying these types of things on impulse will run your bill up without contributing much to your nutrition or to what you have in the house to cook for dinner.

The best way to save on groceries is to be organized and plan ahead. Once a week, read the newspaper grocery store advertisements. Choosing from the best sales, plan what you will eat for the next week and make a grocery list based on your menus. If you do not receive a newspaper, you may be able to see the grocery ads online. The Kroger (www.kroger.com), Albertsons (www.albertsons.com), and Safeway websites (www.safeway.com) have pages where you enter your zip code and can see the weekly ad for your area. In some parts of the country, you can see current sale prices for local grocery stores online at GroceryGuide.com. This website allows you to select the items you wish to buy and print them out as a starting point for making your weekly grocery list. However, in some areas the only stores that are listed on GroceryGuide.com are Walgreens, Rite Aid, etc.

Stick to your grocery list when you shop. Try to do all of your shopping in one weekly trip. Whenever you make a special trip to the store for just one item, you are likely to come home with an entire bag of groceries that you may or may not need. Keep a list of items that are running low and purchase them on your weekly shopping trip. Although you will probably have to do some of your special-diet shopping in a health food store, buy most of your food at the most economical store possible. Store-brand foods are often a better value than national brands. Compare the price per ounce and buy the least expensive brand if the quality is comparable. However, for some items such as paper towel, you may use less of a national brand making that the better buy. For more about grocery shopping and menu planning, see pages 35 to 36 and 45.

Coupon clipping used to be a way to save a little money on food. However, in recent years it seems as if coupons in newspapers are usually for highly processed foods such as frozen dinners, mixes, etc. that those of us with food allergies or gluten intolerance cannot eat. Even if some family members can eat these foods, they are less nutrient dense per dollar than the same foods made at home. Yet, the vigilant shopper may find coupons in grocery store ads for relatively unprocessed foods. Always be discriminating in your use of coupons.

Do It At Home

The more food you prepare at home, the more money you will save on your food budget. Cooking together as a family is also a great bonding experience. Young children will enjoy cooking with you; and as they get older, they will learn skills that will save them money when they are on their own.

My father grew up on a small family-owned vegetable farm in the middle of North Denver during the Great Depression. Several of the few pictures we have of him as a boy are of him and his parents in the field hoeing vegetables together. He often told us how he walked around to their customers' homes pulling his red wagon which was loaded with vegetables to sell. Earning a living was an entire-family experience for him. He always said, "Work hard and work together." While very few families can earn a living together now, we can share our work at home. Letting your children cook with you is a great way to get them started on working hard and working together with others. Giving them chores they must do at home and responsibilities in keeping with their ages teaches them to be dependable hard workers in all areas of their lives. Cooking together also makes cooking more fun for both adults and children.

If you are a "solo" cook, you can still make it enjoyable. Put on your favorite energizing music to listen to while you cook and enjoy the creativity of the cooking experience. While you are cooking, also think about how much money you are saving by cooking at home! For more about how to make cooking easier, see pages 46 to 48 and 30 to 43.

Making good use of your appliances will save you both time and money. With a crock pot you can prepare meals using less-expensive cuts of meat and beans. They will cook all day while you are away and a delicious meal will await you when you get home. Prepare entrées in large batches and freeze part of the batch for future meals. Although the initial investment in a bread machine can seem expensive, it will allow you to make all of your bread at home with very little effort, and the savings will quickly add up to more than the price of the machine. For more about using crock pots, freezers, and bread machines, see pages 37 to 42.

Have Fun With Food

In hard times, it is easy for life to become too serious. However, it is important for both our mental and physical health to lighten up occasionally and have some fun with friends and family. Food allergies or celiac disease can make it difficult to eat out, but there are other kinds of fun we can have that involve food, and this fun can be economical. What makes something fun is not how expensive it is but who you do it with.

For many families, going out for pizza or Chinese food or bringing a pizza or other takeout food home for dinner has been a family treat that is also a way of coping with time pressure. However, with the restrictions of a gluten-free or food allergy diet or with increasing financial pressure, you may have given up this practice. Now is the time to bring back fun with food. Make pizza at home!

Make pizza sauce (recipe on page 178) in large batches and keep it in the freezer. You can make pizza dough that fits your special diet very easily with a bread machine, or make it by hand using the recipes on pages 138 and 179 to 180. Have your children grate cheese and cut up toppings. Mom or Dad may have to stretch the dough out in the pan, but the youngest child can help add the toppings. In addition to having fun making it together, your pizza will be hot and wonderfully delicious and the money you save will add up to a considerable amount over the course of a year.

Picnics are another way to have a great time with friends and family while remaining on a budget. See pages 24 to 25 for more about picnics. During the summer, take a family outing to a local farmers' market. In addition to having fun, you will get some good buys on delicious and nutritious fresh produce.

Waste Not

You have probably heard the old saying, "Waste not, want not." This is certainly true with food. To save money we should try to insure that we do not have to throw food away due to spoilage.

Buying food in large quantities may be a way for large families or people with surplus food storage space to save money. As time goes on, you will come to know the regular prices of the foods you purchase often and will recognize a good sale. If you can afford it, stock up on foods you use often when their prices are significantly reduced. Larger packages of foods may also cost less per ounce. However, do not assume that the larger package always offers the best value. Do the math or read the shelf labels. Surprisingly, more moderately-sized containers are often a better buy. A quantity purchase is not a good deal on perishable foods if they may spoil before they are used up. Even if foods are not perishable, do not buy them in large quantities if they are something that the adults, due to dietary restrictions, cannot eat if the children become tired of them.

The purchase of raw spinach and salad greens is another area where what seems economical may not be. I used to buy fresh spinach in bunches and wash it myself. Unfortunately, I found that, no matter how thoroughly I thought I had dried the spinach, I often could not eat an entire bunch of spinach in salads before it began to spoil. Now I save myself the work of washing and buy plastic clamshells of pre-washed spinach. (The plastic bags of pre-washed spinach also seem more prone to spoilage than the spinach in hard plastic containers). If you are cooking for one or two people and you cannot finish a plastic tub of spinach or salad greens before they spoil, transfer them to a "lettuce keeper" for head lettuce and they will keep longer. See "Sources," page 212, for information on ordering a lettuce keeper.

Maintain inventory control of contents of your refrigerator and freezer. If you know what you have at all times, you can eat your food before it begins to spoil. Buy milk and other perishable dairy products in the quantity you will use before their expiration dates. Do not be shy about picking through the cartons of milk to get one with a better date. Put an E.G.G. (Ethylene Gas Guardian) in the produce drawer(s) of your refrigerator to help protect your produce from spoilage accelerated by ethylene gas. For more about the E.G.G. see page 43.

Take advantage of free food. Chances are you know people who garden and have more zucchini than they can use at the end of the summer. If they want to give you some, take it and fill your freezer with zucchini stew. (See the recipe on page 106. This recipe is the only way I have found to freeze zucchini without it becoming mushy). There is a family in our neighborhood who has an apple tree in their front yard. Every year in the late fall I notice that all the leaves have fallen off the tree but there are still one or two dozen apples hanging and that the ground around the tree is littered with shriveled apples. Every year I think, "What a waste!" Maybe someday if I have grandchildren I'd like to peel apples with, I'll ring this family's doorbell and ask if I can pick their apples in exchange for some homemade applesauce and an apple pie or two. They might appreciate not having the mess to clean up! Peeling apples for pies or sauce with children is a lot of fun if you have the time and an old-fashioned crank apple peeler because they love to turn the crank. Even preschoolers actually can be a real help with this job, and older children enjoy it as well.

Find the Balance

Other ways to save money on food were widely used during the Great Depression such as gardening. If you are a gardener and have the time, go for it! Unfortunately, with gardening, as with many of the suggestions in this book, there is a trade-off between time and money. If you have abundant time, you can peel apples from your own tree and grow your own vegetables. Although my children and I spent a lot of time peeling apples together when they were small, most mothers now hold full-time or part-time jobs, and this way of economizing is not practical. If you are busy, you may need to use some of the commercially prepared foods listed on pages 187 to 208 in spite of the fact that you could save some money by making them yourself. Each of us must find our own personal balance between time and money as we faithfully stay on our diets and try to save both time and money.

Time-Saving Solutions

Time – We could all use more of it. Our lives have become increasingly hectic in recent years. Thankfully, we no longer have to wash our clothes in the stream and our dishes by hand. Besides obvious time-savers such as clothes and dishwashers, many other appliances can save you time if you use them wisely. See pages 37 to 42 and the corresponding recipes chapters for more about using freezers, microwave ovens, crock pots, and bread machines to make your meals and special diet breads with minimal time and effort.

Cooking goes more quickly and easily and can be an enjoyable social experience if you do it with someone else. If you have family members who can assist, enlist their help even if they are children. They will learn to cook by helping you, and in less time than you might expect they will actually be lightening your workload in the kitchen. Helping Dad or Mom cook also helps them learn to be hardworking and responsible.

There are also businesses which can lighten your cooking workload such as restaurants, deli departments of some large health food stores, and commercial food producers. These food producers include not only the makers of frozen entrees, crackers, cookies, breads, and baking mixes, but also the producers of less complex, often single-ingredient foods such as frozen vegetables, canned fruits and vegetables, and pre-washed ready-to-eat salad greens and vegetables.

Bringing Food In and Eating Out

Until the recession began, many families routinely addressed their time problems by eating out or picking up take-out on the way home from work. Now that many Americans find saving money as important as saving time, restaurants and take-out may be an occasional treat rather than a regular routine. However, if you are going to eat out occasionally, you need to know how to do it safely on your diet.

RESTAURANTS

As you read in the last chapter, I rarely eat out, but if your diet allows you to eat fairly freely and you do it in way that avoids exposure to food borne illness, eating out can be a great treat. Celiacs and those with relatively simple food allergies should take a break from cooking to enjoy a meal out when they can afford to.

More and more restaurants are available to cater to celiacs. A friend recently sent me an article from the *New York Times* that featured several gluten-free restaurants in New York City. Even in small towns, people have heard of celiac disease and cater to those who have it. About a month ago, we took our younger son to his second year of college and wanted to spend some time visiting with the family of his best friend so we took them out to lunch at a restaurant which serves buffalo. I was amazed that The Overland Restaurant in Laramie, Wyoming offered me a gluten-free bun for my buffalo burger.

The Gluten Intolerance Group of North American (GIG) offers website help to celiacs who wish to eat out. (See their website at www-gluten-net). They also provide new members with a two-page printed information sheet called "Restaurant Dining: Seven Tips for Staying Gluten-Free" and a wallet-sized restaurant card. This card is meant to be handed to your waiter and lists foods that are allowed and are not allowed on a gluten-free diet. The back of the card lists hidden sources of gluten such as modified food starch, self-basting poultry, and hydrolyzed vegetable protein.

GIG also sponsors the Gluten-Free Restaurant Awareness Program which provides restaurants with information about gluten-free diets and offers food preparation training materials for restaurant staff. Their website lists restaurants that participate in this program at http://www.glutenfreerestaurants.org/find.php. Their online restaurant database is searchable by ZIP code.

The GIG restaurant database is also helpful to those with food allergies who are searching for potential restaurants to try. Restaurants trained by the GIG program are used to special diets and know how not to cross-contaminate foods, so their customers have a better chance of getting the foods they order *plain* and having a meal prepared without butter or bread crumbs from the last customer's meal ending up in the sensitive person's food.

Both celiacs and those with food allergies should take additional steps to achieve a safe dining experience. Call the restaurant a day or more before you plan to visit and ask questions about menu items you would like to order and how they are prepared. If there is only one entrée that you can eat on the menu (as is usually the case for me), ask if they are likely to run out of that food on the day you plan to visit. If the food is something like fresh fish which is not stored in their freezer in abundance at all times, perhaps they can set aside a portion of that food for you.

Other suggestions for safe dining include eating at higher-quality restaurants and timing your meal at a less busy time of day. More expensive restaurants are likely to prepare food to order and can accommodate special requests more easily than chain restaurants. If you go early or late in the dinner or lunch hours, the staff will be able to take more time to listen to your requests and follow them.

Some of the issues you will need to address with your waiter and chef include:

(1) Is this food available *plain?* An explanation of what plain means is in order. It does not just mean without sauces. For meat, it also means not marinated, not tenderized by any means other than pounding with a clean implement, and not pre-basted or injected with butter, hydrolyzed vegetable protein, maltodextrin, or other allergens. Plain turkey is rarely plain because it is difficult to purchase a truly natural turkey; they are almost always injected with something. In addition, prime rib may be cooked rare and brought up to whatever degree of doneness the customer orders by poaching it in a pan of beef broth before serving. This broth is likely to contain a whole list of allergenic or gluten-containing ingredients, but the server may still consider your meat plain because it has not been dressed with gravy. A plain baked potato is not only uncut (specifying that you want your potato uncut helps prevent the addition of butter to the center of the potato) but the skin also has not been rubbed with butter or an allergenic oil before baking. Plain vegetables are boiled with only water and salt, steamed, or baked without anything added. A plain salad is not only free of dressing, but the greens have also not been treated with sulfites to maintain a fresh appearance.

(2) Was there cross-contamination in the preparation of this food? If you order French fries, are they fried in the same vat of oil as battered foods? If they are fried with the same oil that was used for battered fish, your French fries will be contaminated with wheat. If they are fried in a separate vat of oil, you need to ask if it is a kind of oil to which you are allergic. In addition, potato products (including both French fries and hash browns), unless prepared from fresh potatoes, have often been processed with dextrose, dextrins, or starches added by the producer. The restaurant staff may consider them plain, but they were not plain when they came in the back door. The safest way to eat potatoes in a restaurant is to avoid French fries and hash browns and have a baked potato. Even this is not always easy. I once called a restaurant, was told that baked potatoes (the only item I could eat there) were on the lunch menu, got to the restaurant, and found out that baked potatoes were only on the dinner menu. Thankfully, they were willing to microwave a raw potato for me.

Cross-contamination problems are common with other foods also. If you are ordering a salad, will your salad ingredients be chopped on a cutting board contaminated with crouton crumbs from the previous patron's salad? Will your fish be cooked on a grill contaminated with butter from the last order of fish? If you order grilled food, suggest that the chef lay down foil between the grill and your food while cooking it. Unless a restaurant is aware of cross-contamination problems for people on special diets, the same cutting board may be used for the orders of many diners without washing it between different foods, and thus your meal may contain small amounts of many problems foods.

When dining out, even if you have called ahead and the restaurant sounds as if it can meet your needs, it is always wise to carry a few food items in your purse or car just in case. Have a back-up protein supply, such as some home-prepared meat in a cooler or a bag of nuts, in your car. In addition, bring some acceptable crackers and some fresh or dried fruit. Carry a small bottle containing salad dressing that is acceptable on your diet or containing oil for your baked potato in your purse or pocket. Naturally you will put it in a Ziploc™ bag in case it leaks.

If you are dining out and cannot control the selection of the restaurant, eat before you go. Order a cup of tea to sip during the meal, or just sip water and enjoy talking to the other guests. If you cannot have black tea, order tea but specify that you do not want the tea bag (or it may arrive already steeping in your hot water) and bring along an herbal tea bag to use instead.

For more ideas about what foods to order for each meal of the day and tips on dining out from an allergy expert who eats out more than I do, refer to *The Allergy Self-Help Cookbook* by Marjorie H. Jones. For similar advice from the foremost expert on celiac diets and cooking, see *The Gluten-Free Gourmet: Living Well Without Wheat* by Bette Hagman. Both books are listed in the reference section of this book (page 221).

OTHER OPTIONS FOR MEALS AWAY FROM HOME

A picnic is one of the most enjoyable meals to eat away from home. If there are children along, they can leave the table and run around without having to be quiet. The relaxed atmosphere benefits everyone, thus enhancing the eating experience.

Most of the time I prefer a picnic menu that is simple and "disposable." Pack sandwiches for normal family members and guests. If you can eat any type of bread, tortilla, flatbread, or pancake, you can bring a sandwich along for yourself also. If not, some cold meat or bean pate makes a good picnic main dish. (See "Lentil Spread, page 133). Vegetable crudités and healthy chips from the health food store (possibly served with a dip or spread such as lentil spread), a salad with dressing on the side, beverages, and fresh fruit or homemade cookies for dessert round out the meal. We use paper plates and dispose of the trash at the picnic site so there is minimal clean-up when we get home. This is the perfect lunch for a relaxing day in the mountains or at the beach, and since you are in total control of what you eat, an allergic reaction will not spoil your fun.

Occasionally we enjoy the adventure of cooking our lunch at the picnic site. (To appreciate the adventure aspect of this, you should see pictures of us cooking in the rain under an umbrella!) Watching Dad make a fire in the grate is a lot of fun and also offers great picture-taking opportunities. We take hamburgers and two frying pans – a large one for the beef burgers that most of the family and guests will eat and a small one for my game meat burger. We might bring homemade baked beans or other vegetables to warm in the frying pan after the burgers are cooked. Aside from the sandwiches, our usual menu for a cook-out is usually the same as our disposable picnic menu described above.

With microwave oven access available at most workplaces, weekday lunches are easy. If you are on a rotation diet, begin your rotation day at dinner time. Make enough food for the next day's lunch, package it up after dinner, and your lunch will be ready to grab in the morning. If you do not have a microwave oven at your workplace, make extra salad at dinner time and supplement it with some protein which can be eaten cold. This could be the entrée from dinner the night before, other cold meat or fish, or a bag of nuts.

If you are going somewhere and are not sure if you will be home by lunch time, carry nuts and fruit (fresh or dried) along with you in your car. I always have some nuts in my car just in case whatever I have planned for the morning runs longer than expected and I get hungry before I get home.

BRINGING FOOD IN: ASSISTANCE FROM THE DELI

The situation that causes those on special diets the most pressure is that of having nothing planned for dinner when they are on their way home at 5 or 6 p.m. The average person in this quandary can pick up a pizza after work, but this is becoming too expensive for many people to do routinely and is not an option for celiacs and those with food allergies.

The real solution to this problem is to plan ahead as described in the next chapters of this book. However, if you live near a large health food store, some of them have delis that you can visit for a take-out meal. As when you eat in a restaurant, you will have to ask questions, but the deli may have an ingredient label or card for you to read for each food. Before you are in a 5 p.m. crisis situation, visit the deli at a less busy time so you can become familiar with what they have and what you can eat. Be sure to re-check the ingredients before you buy, however! A large health food store near us carries relatively plain roasted free range chickens. My mother-in-law (who could eat anything) used to get their chicken and say that it was better than any chicken she had eaten since she was a girl when all chickens were raised naturally.

In addition, although I do not recommend eating raw items from salad bars anywhere, including in health food stores, a deli salad bar is a good place to get an assortment of pre-cut vegetables to include in a stir-fry or homemade soup. (See page 12 for more about salad bars). As long as the vegetables are adequately cooked before consumption, they should be safe.

Using Convenience Foods

Using commercially prepared foods, especially baked goods, can make it much easier to stay on your diet and lessen your time in the kitchen. The most important thing to remember with these foods is to **read the labels carefully.** If you are just beginning your special diet, set aside an hour or two to visit a large health food store and just read labels. Take a notebook and make a list of items that contain only ingredients which you can eat. Read labels in your grocery store also; the prices for foods you can eat may be lower there. Beware, however, of hidden sources of gluten and food allergens in grocery-store foods. (Although health food store foods tend to be better, they are not immune to containing some hidden allergens). See the "Using Commercially Prepared Foods" section of this book on pages 182 to 186 for a listing of hidden forms of gluten and allergens such as vegetable protein or malt as a hidden form of gluten or wheat, casein or whey as a hidden form of milk, modified food starch as a hidden form of corn, etc. The "Special Diet Resources" section on pages 187 to 208 also provides more ideas than are listed in this chapter for commercially prepared foods that you might be able to use.

FROZEN FOODS

Your health food store freezer is likely to be stocked with a number of gluten-free frozen dinner entrées and many gluten-free baked items such as waffles and breads. Those with multiple food allergies often can find single-grain breads that they can eat in their health food store's freezer. See the "Special Diet Resources" section on pages 188 to 190 for a list of such items that you can purchase from a large store or by mail order. Read the labels each time you shop for these foods to be sure their ingredient lists have not changed.

When shopping for special breads, be aware that some bread labeled yeast-free is not really yeast-free even though no yeast is listed in the ingredients. It may have been prepared by a natural fermentation process, and although no yeast is added, it is leavened by yeast from the air and should be avoided by those with yeast allergy. If the bread is truly yeast-free, the ingredient list will contain baking soda and/or other leavening ingredients.

GLUTEN-FREE AND WHEAT-FREE BAKED GOODS

Commercial food producers have risen to the challenge of baking for the celiac diet. Our health food store carries many varieties of gluten-free baking mixes for everything from corn bread to chocolate cakes. If you are a celiac with additional food sensitivities, be sure to read the labels on the baking mixes carefully; there is a good chance that you will be able to use at least some of these mixes. However, to prevent rice sensitivity, you may wish to vary the grain or grain alternative you eat from day to day and not use rice-based baking mixes exclusively. For recipes made with grains other than rice, see the baking recipes on pages 135 to 151 and pages 156 to 170 of this book and also the recipes in *Gluten-Free Without Rice* as described on the last pages of this book.

Your health food store also probably carries a large variety of gluten-free crackers, cookies, cereals, and snacks. Again read the labels to check for ingredients that may cause you problems if you have other sensitivities, and do not rely solely on rice. As an added caution, re-read the labels of your favorite brands each time you purchase them to be sure the ingredients have not changed.

For a list of commercially prepared baked goods that you might be able to use, see "Special Diet Resources" on pages 187 to 208. Many of these items can be purchased by mail order if you live in an area without a large heath food store. If you have Internet access and would like to shop at Vitamin Cottage Natural Grocers, the health food store where I shop, visit www.naturalgrocers.com. They have a Shop-by-Diet search tool that will help celiacs find the hundreds of gluten-free and allergen-free products they carry. Those with food allergies can also shop by diet to avoid individual food allergens. If you are allergic to a number of foods, you may be able to find items that are free of all of your problem foods by reading the ingredient lists (click on "back of the bag") for foods you find by searching for one of your problem foods.

Another way to find reliable producers of additional gluten-free foods is to check the gluten-free product listing on the Gluten Intolerance Group (GIG) website at www.gluten.net. If you do not have Internet access, new members of the GIG receive a printed handout which, at the time of this writing, contains about 120 companies that produce gluten-free foods.

CANNED VEGETABLE, BEEF, AND CHICKEN BROTH

Most commercially prepared broths are a land mine of chemicals and allergens. (For a list of some of these strange ingredients, see pages 58 to 59). However, at the time of this writing, there a few broths which are made with only meat, and/or poultry (or their pure extracts), vegetables, water, salt, and spices. See pages 202 to 204 for a listing of some of these broths. They are convenient to have on hand for throwing together a quick soup or for making some of the main dish recipes in this book.

VEGETABLES AND FRUITS

While usually not thought of as convenience foods, frozen, canned, and pre-washed and cut fresh fruits and vegetables definitely can save you a lot of time in the kitchen. Compare shelling peas to purchasing a bag of them frozen! Or think about using frozen or pre-cut and washed fresh broccoli instead of cutting a large stem of broccoli into bite-size pieces yourself. Although freshly picked vegetables have the highest levels of nutrients, those that are frozen soon after picking retain more nutrients than vegetables which have been stored several days in transit or in your refrigerator.

You can save time by using pre-washed salad greens also. I remember my dad's lettuce and spinach grown in his garden. They were incredibly delicious freshly picked and certainly had the maximum amounts of nutrients, but it was a major chore to wash all the dirt and bugs out of them using salt in the first wash and then using several changes of water. Unless you grow your own salad vegetables, if you are pressed for time, pre-washed bagged salads certainly are handy. The recipes in this book make use of convenience produce whenever possible.

Canned vegetables do not have the crisp textures and flavors of fresh or frozen vegetables, so I avoid using most of them, with a few exceptions such as those below. If you do use them, read the labels carefully for ingredients such as sugar, corn syrup, and flavor enhancers that may contain gluten. The stroganoff recipe in this book (page 69) calls for either fresh or canned mushrooms because using canned saves time on cleaning and slicing mushrooms. I find canned tomatoes indispensable for soups and use tomato paste, sauce, and puree in Italian cook-ing. Be aware, however, that tomato products require diligent label-reading. If you think a certain brand is all right, be sure to read it every time you buy it anyway. I was recently shocked to find that a brand of plain tomato sauce that my grand-mother used years ago and that is made by a producer with an Italian name had added sugar and a number of other ingredients to their sauce. The ingredient list of a store brand of Italian-style tomato paste includes tomato paste, water, sugar, salt, spices, Romano cheese, soy oil, hydrolyzed corn protein, wheat gluten, soy protein, garlic, torula yeast, and natural flavors. A person with a sensitivity to anything would be likely to react to something in that tomato paste! A national brand of chopped tomatoes had high fructose corn syrup in all of their flavored or variety canned tomatoes. The lesson is – always read labels carefully!

If you have difficulty finding plain canned vegetables or all-tomato canned tomato products, check the salt-free versions of each brand. These tend to be free of other potentially problematic ingredients in addition to salt. Organic canned vegetables are also more likely to be plain. If you are highly sensitive to yeast and cannot eat canned tomato products in general due to yeast, see *The Ultimate Food Allergy Cookbook and Survival Guide* for sauce recipes made from fresh tomatoes.

Fresh locally produced fruit is always the most delicious, but there are times when canned and frozen fruit is a real time-saver. I haven't cut up a fresh pineapple in years because pineapple canned in its own juice is so convenient. If you are making a dessert with berries when they are out of season, frozen berries are the thing to use. To save time on washing, stemming and sorting, you also might use them when fresh berries are available. For apple pie or apple crisp, canned peeled and sliced apples save a lot of time. Read the label and be sure what you are buying is only apples and water. You do not want to mistakenly purchase apple pie filling made with sugar, high fructose corn syrup and thickeners that might contain gluten.

Frozen, canned, and refrigerated fruit and vegetable juices are so common, economical, and convenient that you must be a dedicated juicer to make your own juice. In addition to consuming commercially prepared fruit juices plain, you might enjoy using them to make tasty and nutritious beverages that are a good substitute for sodas. Just mix some fruit juice or thawed fruit juice concentrate with carbonated water, add a little ice and a straw to make it special, and your kids (or you) will not be tempted to reach for a can of pop. See the fruit juice soda recipe on page 174.

By making use of help from others, especially commercial food producers, you can stay on your diet with less work. See the "Special Diet Resources" section of this book on pages 187 to 208 for more ideas of convenience foods that you can use. The "Using Commercially Prepared Foods" section on pages 182 to 186 contains as a list of hidden sources of allergenic ingredients to refer to when you read labels.

Cooking with Ease

Cooking does not have to be complicated. If you simplify, organize, use the right recipes, and put your appliances to work efficiently, you can save money and spend less time in the kitchen than you may have spent in the past. You can cook with ease. As you get more used to cooking, it becomes second nature and you may come to appreciate it as a creative, grounding activity.

Shopping and Stocking

THE FOODS YOU NEED

The first thing you have to do when you cook is shop for the ingredients that you will need. If you have a well-stocked kitchen, your weekly shopping will be simplified because most of your shopping list will be fresh items for the next week's meals. Keeping your pantry and freezer well stocked with the ingredients you use routinely will make cooking easier to manage all around.

When you are just starting with a special diet, your pantry or cupboards may need a major overhaul. If you are too busy to bake routinely for non-allergic family members, consider cleaning out the wheat flour, gluten- or allergen-containing mixes, and other ingredients that you can no longer eat; buy your family's normal baked goods already made. If you will use these wheat-containing ingredients to bake on special occasions and your pantry is full, perhaps they can be moved to another place such as the basement for storage. Then stock your pantry with items such as these:

Many types of flours and grains or grain alternatives: If you are on a rotation diet, you should have a different flour and grain or grain alternative for each day of your rotation. Hopefully you have at least four or five that you can eat! If you are on a gluten-free diet, also consider expanding the variety of flours and grains that you eat and possibly eating them in a rotated pattern with a few days off before you eat the same grain again. This should keep you from becoming sensitive to rice. For more about gluten-free cooking with grains other than rice, see *Gluten-Free Without Rice* as described on the last pages of this book.

Baking mixes: If you are on a gluten-free diet and can use the many baking mixes found in your health food store, keep some of your favorites on hand. If you have allergies but can use some of the gluten-free mixes, you might wish to have a keep a few in your pantry as well. Although most baking mixes are based on rice, Chebe™ bread mixes are made with manioc (cassava) flour. You must add an egg or two to each of their mixes, and some of them also call for milk products. If you can eat eggs, you may want to get some Chebe™ bread mix at a health food store or online to add more variety to your diet. (See "Resources," page 195 to purchase Chebe™ mixes). Although mixes may save you time, baked good are considerably less expensive if you start from flour and other ingredients. Using simple recipes such as those in this book, you will spend five to ten minutes more baking from scratch than with a mix. If you make larger batches and need to bake less often, you can come out ahead on both time and money by baking from scratch. Also, overuse of rice or cassava (or any food) may lead to sensitivity to these grains. (See pages 10 to 11 for more about rice sensitivity). It is good to have a few mixes on hand for when you are really pressed for time, but baking from scratch is best for both health and economy. See pages 61 to 64 for ways to make baking easier.

Other essential pantry staples include **grain products** such as **pasta**, hot or cold **cereals**, **crackers** that fit your diet, and healthy **grain snacks** such as popcorn, wheat-free pretzels, and sugar-free, gluten- or allergen-free cookies. If you have multiple food allergies, there might not be much in the way of cereals, snacks, and crackers that you can purchase, so you should keep a supply of homemade cookies, crackers, and other baked goods for each day of your rotation diet in your freezer instead. To make healthy popocorn, see the recipe on page 175.

Starches are useful ingredients to have in your pantry for thickening. If you are not allergic to corn, cornstarch is easy to find at the grocery store. Health food stores carry tapioca flour or arrowroot which are used in baking as well as for thickening. Authentic Foods™ and Bob's Red Mill™ brands of tapioca starch and arrowroot are often found on the baking aisle. Granulated (or minute) tapioca can be purchased at the grocery store and used to thicken pie fillings, puddings, and stews. For thickening salad dressings and other foods without cooking them, QuickThick™ and ThickenUp™, which are a type of cornstarch, are very easy to use. These thickeners for liquids, which are used by stroke victims and people who have trouble swallowing thin liquids, may be purchased at a pharmacy or online. (See "Sources," page 214).

Leavening ingredients are essential pantry staples for baking. Those on strict allergy rotation diets often use a combination of **baking soda** and **unbuffered vitamin C** powder or crystals to avoid eating the starch in baking powder every day. The vitamin C used for leavening must be unbuffered. This means it does not contain minerals such as calcium, magnesium, etc. which make it less acidic.

See "Sources," page 211 for information about purchasing hypoallergenic cassava source unbuffered vitamin C.

Baking soda is an essential pantry staple for leavening non-yeast baked goods. It is also handy to have for other uses such as absorbing odors in the refrigerator, freshening the garbage disposal, or for other household cleaning.

If you use **baking powder**, be sure to choose a brand which does not contain aluminum and, if you are a celiac, which is gluten-free. Bob's Red Mill™ baking powder is certified gluten-free and is aluminum-free. Like most baking powder, it contains cornstarch. If you are allergic to corn but can eat potatoes, buy Feather-weight™ baking powder which contains potato starch instead of cornstarch. It is also free of aluminum, gluten and sodium. Most health food stores carry Feather-weight™ baking powder, or see "Sources," page 211.

Yeast does not belong in the pantry for long-term storage but is included here with other leavening agents because it is an essential baking supply if you make yeast leavened baked goods. If you make an occasional loaf of bread or wheat-free pizza, buy individual packets of yeast at your grocery store. Keep these packets in the refrigerator. However, if you bake often, it is more economical to purchase yeast in larger quantities. Red Star Active Dry and SAF instant yeast are very eco-nomical in one pound bags. They cost as little as $5 for a pound of yeast and are vacuum sealed so they can be stored in the pantry until the bag is opened. Once you open the package, put a little of the yeast in a jar in the refrigerator and store the rest in the freezer. When your jar is empty, do not allow the frozen yeast to thaw, but instead pour a small amount into the jar and put the rest back into the freezer. You can make many, many loaves of bread with just a few dollars worth of yeast if you treat your yeast this way.

Sweeteners are also usually stored in the pantry. The most common sweetener in the average pantry is sugar. The dessert recipes in this book, with the excep-tion of the chocolate brownies recipe, do not contain sugar so you may not need sugar. Instead, your pantry may contain **Fruit Sweet**™ (or equivalent sweeteners also made Wax Orchards such as Pear Sweet™ or Grape Sweet™) or **honey** to use in desserts instead. Fruit Sweet™ can be stored at room temperature until it is opened. After that, store it in the refrigerator. Honey can be stored in the pantry even after it is opened. Other sweeteners you may find in a sugar-free pantry include **date sugar**, which is ground dried dates, and **rice sweeteners.** Celiacs should be aware that brown rice syrup almost always contains barley or enzymes from barley and therefore is not gluten-free.

In addition to containing fructose rather than sucrose, some fruit sweeteners are lower in calories for the amount of sweetness delivered. Fruit Sweet™, Pear Sweet™, and Grape Sweet™ are sweeter than sugar but have 30% fewer calories.

They also contain fiber and minerals which have been refined out of table sugar. These sweeteners have been featured in the American Dietetic Association's catalogue for use by people with diabetes.

An intriguing "new" sweetener that you may have in your pantry is **agave** which comes from a plant in the yucca family as does **aguamiel**. These sweeteners can be stored at room temperature after they are opened. You will find agave near the honey in your health food store and can use it like honey in cooking. Agave is low on the glycemic index, 90% fructose, and sweeter than sugar so less is needed. Its flavor is neutral, so it tastes delicious in all types of desserts. It will be featured in a new dessert cookbook in 2009. For more about agave, see page 57.

Frozen fruit juice concentrates are also wonderful for sweetening desserts and are included here even though you will keep them in the freezer until you are about to use them. Several hours or the night before you plan to bake, move the fruit juice to the refrigerator to thaw. If you will be baking often with a certain fruit juice after it is thawed, you may store it in the refrigerator until the next time you bake.

Some **oils** and **fats** can be stored in your pantry. However, if you use them slowly, storing them in your refrigerator will delay rancidity. The best oil for cooking with moderate or high heat, such as sautéing, is olive oil because it does not break down or become a damaged fat when heated. Ghee, or clarified butter, can be stored at room temperature in your pantry and is another good fat for cooking at moderate to high heat because it is a saturated fat. Oils high in essential fatty acids, such as canola oil or walnut oil, are best used for salads and on cooked vegetables. Flax oil is the best nutritional oil for providing essential fatty acids and also can be used in salad dressings. Since it is quite fragile, it should be refrigerated.

Dry beans are essential residents of a well-stocked pantry. Keep some kidney beans for chili, and stock mixed beans, black beans, lentils, or split peas for soup. Because beans plus a grain constitute a complete protein, they are an excellent substitute for meat in your diet. Serve one of the many easy crock pot bean soup recipes in this book (pages 91 to 95) with bread or crackers and you will receive superior nutrition while saving money. Bean soups can cook all day while you are away, and you will come home to a delicious dinner, ready to eat, and leftover soup to freeze for future meals. If your family is not quite ready for a vegetarian dinner, try "Economy Chili" (page 97) to stretch your meat dollars and stock up your freezer for future meals.

Having your pantry stocked with **canned goods** can save you many an emergency trip to the grocery store. Canned and aseptically packaged products can be stored at room temperature until you open them.

Fruit juice or water-packed canned fruits are delicious. They can be handy additions to any meal or the makings of a great dessert. If you want to make an apple crisp in the blink of an eye, keep some water-packed canned apples such as Mussleman's™ apples in your pantry. Read the ingredient list on the fruit cans before you purchase them and avoid those with added sugar or corn syrup. Small cups of unsweetened or apple juice-sweetened applesauce are great snacks to keep in your pantry.

Fresh and frozen **vegetables** are usually tastier than most canned vegetables, but having a few cans of vegetables in your pantry might save you a trip to the grocery store sometime. As with fruits, read the ingredient list on vegetable cans before you purchase them and avoid those with added sugar or corn syrup.

Tomato products are essential pantry staples. If you have room and want to save money, stock up on diced canned tomatoes, tomato sauce, tomato paste and tomato puree when they are on sale and have them on hand at all times. Many people like to keep jarred pasta sauces in their pantry because these sauces can be used to whip up a quick meal, and gluten- and allergen-free sauces can be purchased at health food stores. Since our family is Italian, we make our own sauce and keep it in the freezer. Don't let that discourage you from stocking pasta sauce in your own pantry! Be sure to read labels carefully on tomato products, however. See pages 28 to 29 for more about ingredients you might find in them.

Canned dried beans are useful pantry staples. Keep a couple of cans of kidney beans on hand to make chili in a hurry, or keep a variety of beans for side dishes such as three bean salad. Since many brands of canned beans contain sugar or corn syrup, you must read the can labels. However, salt-free varieties and some of the natural or organic brands such as Westbrae™ brand are sugar-free.

Canned broth can be useful to have in your pantry for main dish recipes and as a base for quick soups. Many broths contain sugar or gluten-derived products such as monosodium glutamate (MSG) and other additives. (See pages 58 to 59 for more about this). Natural canned broths that are gluten- and allergen-free are listed on pages 202 to 204.

Condiments such as mayonnaise, pickles, catsup, and mustard are essential residents in the pantry of anyone who likes hamburgers. Read the labels and avoid such allergenic ingredients as eggs and gluten-containing malt or grain vinegar. Choose a fruit-juice sweetened catsup such as Westbrae™ brand rather than a brand made with sugar or corn syrup. Salsa is another condiment you might want to have on hand for "Ground Beef Enchilada Casserole," page 79. If you are allergic to yeast, you will need to avoid all of these because they contain vinegar. Celiacs must read condiment labels carefully to avoid malt or grain vinegar. For recipes to make these condiments without vinegar, see *The Ultimate Food Allergy Cookbook and Survival Guide* which is described on the last pages of this book.

Keep **sandwich fixings** such as a variety of natural nut butters and all-fruit jam or jelly in your pantry. If you are allergic to peanuts, try cashew, almond, macadamia, or other natural nut butters. All are a great source of essential fatty acids. If you like fish salad sandwiches, a can or two of tuna or salmon is good to have on hand.

Other items you may want to stock in your pantry include unsweetened baking chocolate, cocoa or carob, coffee, tea, raisins and other dry fruit, unsweetened coconut, carob or chocolate chips, non-fat dry milk or dry goat milk, cooking wine, wine vinegar, and **seasonings** such as salt, pepper, cinnamon, nutmeg, cloves, ginger, vanilla extract, basil, oregano, thyme, bay leaves, chili powder, dry mustard, and paprika.

ROUTINE GROCERY SHOPPING TRIPS

With organization and planning, major weekly grocery shopping trips do not have to be a chore or very expensive. You might even be able to replace a weekly trip with a slightly larger biweekly trip and an in-between-week run for produce and dairy products. Unscheduled trips to the store to "just get a few things" can be eliminated. This will reduce the total amount of time you spend waiting in checkout lines and has the added benefit for your grocery budget of curbing impulse spending.

For the best shopping experience, try to shop at a time of the day and week when the store is not overly crowded. Thus you can zip through the aisles quickly and avoid long lines for checkout. Always eat a meal before you shop. If you go shopping when you are hungry, the foods you cannot eat will call out to you! There is no need to make yourself feel deprived in this way. In addition, hunger will make you more easily tempted to buy the high-priced goodies (if your family members can eat them) which are so attractively displayed in prominent places. I routinely follow up my weekly trip to the grocery store with a trip to the health food store. Knowing that I can get an inexpensive "legal treat" at my final stop prevents me from feeling deprived when I see displays of foods I cannot eat at the grocery store.

Making shopping easier and more economical requires advance planning. Read the weekly newspaper grocery store and health food store advertisements and plan menus for the next week or two. If you are on a rotation diet, what you will eat each day may be pre-determined. If not, you can save money by choosing from the best sales when you plan menus. See page 17 for more about shopping the grocery store ads.

Keep a spiral notebook or steno pad in your kitchen to use for your weekly grocery lists. If you are on a rotation diet, there will be certain foods you purchase every week. Write those on each page of the notebook for several weeks at once. If family members need certain staples every week (milk, lettuce, etc.) write those on each page of the notebook as well. When you read the grocery ads and plan menus, add the foods required for the week's menus to your basic list on that week's note-book page. When you notice you are beginning to run low on staple foods that you have stocked in your pantry or freezer, add them to the grocery list immediately. If you wait until you completely run out of these foods, you will find yourself inter-rupting your baking time to make a special trip to the store "just for baking soda" someday. If you come home with more than just baking soda, you may have blown your grocery budget as well as having spent time at the store unnecessarily.

Stick to your grocery list when you shop; it will save you money and keep you from getting distracted and forgetting something important. If you are very orga-nized, you might even want to designate certain parts of the page on your shopping list for certain categories of foods and gear these categories to the layout of your favorite store. Then follow a pre-set pattern on your trip through the store. I start in the part of the store where room-temperature items are found and pick up paper products, canned goods, bottled beverages, etc. first. Then I shop for heavy perish-able items such as dairy products. Next I pick up meat, poultry and seafood. I shop for produce towards the end of the trip so I do not smash produce by putting heavy items on top of the tomatoes! Finally, I buy frozen juices, fruits, and vegetables.

If you are shopping for less-familiar types of produce as you begin an allergy diet, see the chapter about shopping in *Easy Cooking for Special Diets* (as described on the last page of this book) or search the Internet to learn how to choose produce that you haven't purchased before. Have a learning experience rather than letting a lack of knowledge keep you from trying a new vegetable that can add to your nutrition and round out a rotation diet.

Use Your Appliances and Gadgets

We have many advantages over our grandmothers or great-grandmothers when it comes to getting things done in the kitchen – self-cleaning ovens, dishwashers, microwave ovens, bread machines, freezers, crock pots, and the list goes on. Of course, like the rest of the adult population today, most mothers also have outside-the-home work. Some of our ancestors, such as my paternal grandmother, worked in the farm fields in addition to doing their inside chores. I don't know how she managed it all without a clothes washer and dryer (she washed clothes in a tub with a wash board and hung them to dry) or the modern kitchen appliances listed below. These appliances and gadgets save a lot of time and money and make life much easier. Although it does cost money to purchase these appliances initially, if they make it possible for you to prepare most of your food at home rather than eating out or purchasing many commercially prepared foods, the net result will be tremendous financial savings over time.

FREEZERS

A freezer is the most useful appliance we have for maximizing the efficiency of our time in the kitchen. By properly using freezer space, we can save ourselves work by cooking things in large batches and freezing part of each batch for future meals. If you are on a rotation diet for your food allergies and are not able to use most commercially made baked goods, you should keep a good supply of the baked goods you need for each rotation day in your freezer. It's rough to wake up and have no bread type of food to eat for breakfast unless you bake! Plus, who has time to bake before starting the day? Thankfully, the small freezer most of us have in our refrigerators is large enough to make rotation possible without a daily crisis.

First of all, rid your freezer of the food that you really don't need to store long-term. Eliminate everything that is old and have non-allergic family members eat as much of the rest of the food as possible. If you are limited to the freezer space at the top of your refrigerator, there is no need to keep several flavors of ice cream, a dozen packages of vegetables, or anything that you will probably never eat. Do not store more frozen vegetables, juices, or other items than you will use between major grocery shopping trips. For most of us, this means you need to get your stockpile of frozen produce and commercially made frozen foods down to a one-week supply. Neatly stack those foods on one side of the freezer section of your refrigerator and use the rest of the space for your homemade special foods.

When you make main dishes or bake bread, muffins, or crackers, prepare large batches and freeze what you do not eat immediately. To save freezer space, freeze serving-sized portions of entrées in Seal-a-Meal™ bags, zippered plastic bags, or rectangular freezer containers, clearly labeling them with the all the ingredients (in case you later find you must change your rotation) and date. If your freezer meals are packaged in uniformly sized and shaped containers, you can get a lot of them into the top freezer section of a refrigerator. Cook on the weekends and take things out of the freezer on weekdays. Keep your freezer organized (for example, assign foods from each rotation day a certain location in the freezer) so you can find what you need to eat on each rotation day quickly. If you are hungry and it is too hard to find something, you may get frustrated and eat something to which you are allergic instead.

Nearly emptying your freezer of the foods you now have in it may seem daunting. However, once you have tried using your freezer in the way described above, you will discover that this is a good system not only for people on special diets but also for anyone who eats mostly homemade foods, as illustrated by the following story.

My older son is a third year graduate student, and although he is not on a special diet except for three weeks a year around the time of his annual LDA shot (see page 49 for more about this), he does all of his own cooking and rarely eats out. He is used to homemade bread so makes his own hamburger buns and bread using a bread machine. When he makes buns, he makes a large batch and freezes most of them. The last two years his usual routine for making dinners was to make a large batch of something on the weekend and eat it every night for the next week. On Saturday, he follows a three generation family tradition and has a hamburger for dinner.

I encouraged him to use the freezer section of his refrigerator for entrées in the way described above for the last two years. Admittedly, since his old refrigerator had a large ice maker and no shelf (which encouraged anything stacked on something else to fall out onto the floor every time the freezer was opened), I can see why it was not easy to take my advice.

This year he is living in a house with two other guys instead of with one apartment-mate. The other guys were there first and had the freezer well filled, so there was not much room in the freezer section of their kitchen refrigerator for his hamburger buns for Saturday nights. Therefore he purchased a 5 cubic foot chest freezer for less than $200 which he keeps in the garage off the kitchen. The first week he had his freezer he told me it contained ice cubes left over from a large bag of ice purchased for a picnic. Gradually, as he made large batches of chili (see page 97 for his variation of my recipe), burritos, and other entrées, he put meal-sized portions of them into his freezer. This week he made chicken enchiladas for dinner, but a batch makes only enough to last him for three dinners. He told me this works out well now that he has a good assortment of entrees in his freezer. He plans to takes one frozen entrée out each weeknight after the enchiladas are gone. Since variety in the diet is the basis of good nutrition, I am glad that he is using his freezer in a way that is moving him towards more variety in his meals. Not eating the same thing for five or six nights in a row has to be more satisfying too!

OVENS – MICROWAVE AND CONVENTIONAL

Microwave ovens were developed to save time. Now that we've had them for almost three decades, few of us feel we could live without them. The freezer system for entrees described on the previous pages works best when you have a microwave oven to heat the entrée taken from the freezer. Although microwave ovens are not usually the best method for cooking main dishes, they are the best way to reheat most foods. They are also good for cooking vegetables. You can use your microwave to cook vegetables while your main dish is cooking on the stove top or broiling in the oven. If your family does not like the taste or texture of microwaved potatoes as well as they like conventionally baked potatoes, see the recipes for "Nuke-n-Bake Potatoes" and other microwave-plus-conventionally cooked vegetables on pages 106 to 108. For more about microwaving vegetables and a few other microwave recipes, see pages 105 and 108 to 112.

A conventional oven, especially if you have a time-bake feature, can be used to cook a whole meal easily at one time. Just bake the entrée, a grain or starchy vegetable (such as white potatoes, sweet potatoes, or winter squash), a non-starchy vegetable, and dessert all together as an "oven meal." Put the components of the meal in your oven on time bake when you will be gone for a few hours or start them in the mid-afternoon when you will be at home and let things cook while you work.* At dinner time, you will not have to spend any more time in the kitchen before dinner than it takes to make a salad. For oven vegetable and side dish recipes, see pages 80 to 85. For recipes for entrées, see pages 74 to 79. Simple desserts that can bake for a flexible amount of time are good as part of an oven meal. These recipes are found on pages 154 to 155.

*Note: Do not put a time-bake meal in the oven before you leave for work in the morning. It is unsafe to leave raw meat at room temperature (such as in the oven) for more than an hour or so before the time-bake feature turns the oven on.

CROCK POTS

Crock pots are my favorite kitchen appliance. After you have been gone all day, they make your house smell good. When you walk in the door, a warm feeling surrounds you because you can tell that dinner is ready and will be delicious.

Crock pots are inexpensive, last nearly forever, save money on groceries, and can make your life much easier. You can prepare ingredients in the evening, start your dinner in just a few minutes the next morning and leave the crock pot to cook all day while you work. When you get home, your dinner is ready for you to enjoy. A 3-quart crock pot costs $20 or less at a discount department store at the time of this writing. With a 5 or 6-quart crock pot, which you can get for just a few dollars more, you can make large batches of foods and stock your freezer for several meals. The long, slow cooking of a crock pot is ideal for tenderizing game meat or inexpensive cuts of meat and making delicious soups and stews from beans and less expensive cuts of meat.

Here are a few tips for using a crock pot. To have the contents of the crock pot heat up in an optimal amount of time, it should be about ⅔ to ¾ full. If you fill the pot more than this it requires a longer time to heat up and thus longer to cook. I admit to filling my crock pot nearly full on a regular basis, so the recipes in this book have cooking times that account for the pot being nearly full when it is turned on. If your pot is full and you will be home, you can shorten the warm-up time by cooking on high for the first hour or two of the cooking time and then turning it down to low. Some crock pots have a convenient feature that cooks on high for an hour and then turns the pot to low automatically.

There are times to look in and times not to lift the lid of a crock pot. Don't peek in the crock pot repeatedly because it allows heat to escape. Lifting the lid requires time for the pot to come back to the desired temperature each time and may lengthen the cooking time. A few of the recipes in this book say to stir the pot during cooking, and the cooking times account for this. However, you should lift the lid at the end of the cooking time if you want to thicken the sauce in a crock pot recipe. Turn the temperature to high and cook it with the lid off or ajar for the last half hour of cooking time.

For crock pot recipes, see pages 86 to 95 and 97 to 102.

BREAD MACHINES

At an allergy cooking class I taught a few years ago I was asked, "Do you have any recommendations for people who are on a special diet and don't want to spend a lot of time baking?" My immediate reply was, "Get a bread machine!" If you must make most of your own baked goods from scratch, and especially if you can eat yeast breads, a bread machine is an incredible time-saver.

Some wheat-free yeast breads such as spelt, kamut, rye, and egg-containing rice breads can be made with almost any bread machine. Others such as oat, barley, egg-free rice, buckwheat, amaranth, and quinoa can be made using a programmable machine on which you can control the last rising time. For detailed help in choosing a machine that fits your needs, see *Easy Breadmaking for Special Diets* as described on the last pages of this book.

For a quick answer to the question, "What machine should I buy?" at the time of this writing, the only truly programmable machine currently on the market that works well for non-wheat breads is the Zojirushi BBCC-X20. It's a bit pricey (around $200) but it and the previous similar models have all been excellent machines for special diet breads, as well as for making great wheat bread. Zojirushi machines are well made and last a long time. If you consider the price of store-bought alternative yeast breads, you will recoup your investment in a matter of a few months. My Zojirushi BBCC-V20 is getting noisy but still going strong after about ten years of heavy use. Because I must keep up on bread machines that are the best for people with food allergies, I also have a Zojirushi BBCC-X20. It is very similar to the V20 except you can store programs for three custom cycles rather than one and have the option of turning of the pre-heat part of any cycle. To purchase the Zojirushi BBCC-X20 machine by mail order from the King Arthur Flour Bakers Catalogue, see "Sources," page 212. This machine is also available from Amazon.com and some large houseware stores.

If you can eat spelt or rice and eggs and do not expect to use your bread machine only often, the Sunbeam 5891 bread machine may provide you with an economical alternative to the Zojirushi bread machine. My friend Linda Bonvie, coauthor of *Chemical-Free Kids* and *Chemical-Free Kids: The Organic Sequel,* owns a Sunbeam 5891 which she uses often and really likes. This machine costs about $70 at the time of this writing. Although it is advertised as programmable, the only thing that you can program is the delayed-start timer. You cannot program a shorter last rise, which is needed for many gluten-free breads. However, if you can eat spelt bread or egg-containng rice bread, this machine will meet your needs and is reliable and inexpensive. You will be able to make pizza easily at home using this machine, and if you do that once a month, it will pay for itself in about six months.

Yeast-free breads and cakes can be made in some bread machines. A few of the bread machines on the market have a cake or quick bread cycle which will work to make yeast-free allergy or gluten-free breads. The type of cycle needed mixes for just a few minutes and then immediately bakes the bread. (The Zojirushi BBCC-X20 has such a cycle; the cake cycle on the Sunbeam 5891 does not mix and thus does not save you work). If you are on a yeast-free diet and purchasing a bread machine, be careful that you are getting a machine that will work for allergy or celiac diet yeast-free bread. For more information about making yeast-free breads using a bread machine, see *Easy Breadmaking for Special Diets* as described on the last pages of this book.

A bread machine may not be a money and time-saving investment for you if you are on a yeast-free diet and/or plan to eat muffins, crackers, cookies and other small baked items most of the time with yeast-free or yeast-leavened bread only the occasional treat. Non-yeast breads are easily mixed by hand. In addition, if you are on a yeast-free diet, the recipes you will need will be different than for those who can eat yeast. You can find basic yeast-free as well as yeast-containing allergy bread machine recipes, hand-mixed versions of the same recipes, and recipes for muffins, crackers, etc. in *The Ultimate Food Allergy Cookbook and Survival Guide* as described on the last pages of this book. If you can tolerate yeast and want basic bread recipes (both yeast leavened and yeast-free) plus many more creative bread recipes and bread making and bread machine advice, see *Easy Breadmaking for Special Diets,* as described on the last pages of this book.

HAND BLENDERS

There are some appliances that do a great job, but they are so large that they will not all fit on your counter. Storing them in closets or cupboards makes them a hassle to haul out and use, and their size also usually means that they must be washed by hand. Food processors, blenders, and electric mixers fall into this category for me; they are almost more trouble than they are worth. They also can be expensive to purchase.

A handy inexpensive substitute for these appliances is a hand blender. This versatile little item can overcome lumps in gravy or pudding, make low-fat yet thick salad dressings, puree soup, and at times will seem like your best friend in the kitchen. Inexpensive hand blenders can be purchased at discount department stores for less than $20 at the time of this writing. Since hand blenders are small, they are easily stored in a kitchen cabinet and are easy to wash. On some (the more expensive models) the blending blade section detaches from the handle and can be put in the dishwasher. On the cheaper ones you can just swish the end with the blending blade in soapy water and then rinse it. Like many other cooks, I would be lost without a hand blender.

THE E.G.G. ™

The E.G.G.™ (ethylene gas guardian) is a refrigerator gadget that can save you both money and time. About three months ago I purchased my first E.G.G.™ package, which is a set of two plastic eggs containing potassium permanganate, a substance that absorbs ethylene gas. The instructions say to put one egg in each produce drawer of your refrigerator, and it will help produce stay fresh longer. These little things work! Yesterday I removed the remains of a very old bag of radishes that I purchased when we had guests for dinner nearly two months ago. They were not rotten, although there were a few brown spots on two of the radishes.

If you have planned a menu to include a certain fresh produce item, it is nice to reach into the fruit or vegetable drawer and find that produce is still fresh and edible. These little eggs can keep your menu plans from being disrupted by rotten food. In addition to saving you money on spoiled produce, they will also save you some refrigerator clean-up time. To purchase them, see "Sources," page 209.

YOU'RE ALMOST THERE

This chapter contains a lot of advice about what to have on hand to cook economically and with ease – both food items stocked in your cupboards or pantry and freezer and the appliances and gadgets that will help you with the work. As you gather these items and prepare to cook, organize your kitchen for efficiency. Put the silverware and dishes near the table, if possible. Put the utensils you use for cooking near the stove. Arrange your panty and freezer so similar foods are grouped together in an organized fashion. If your kitchen is organized well, you will not have to spend time searching for something when you want to cook. If you organize your kitchen for efficiency now, it will save you much time later.

When you have followed the advice in this chapter, you are primed to cook. The next chapter will address some wider issues, and then you will be completely ready to go.

Organization, Planning, and Other Money and Time Savers

The kitchen is organized. Now it's time organize yourself and your life. Many of you, I'm sure, already make good use of your day-timers. If you do, please do not be offended that at the basic organization advice below.

GENERAL ORGANIZATION AND TIME MANAGEMENT

Often when people learn they have celiac disease or food allergies, they are so overwhelmed that inertia sets in. This doesn't help. They need to get organized and move on to the things necessary to improve their health. This section of the book tells how to do that at the most basic level.

When you start a special diet, you will probably be adding the work of cooking most of your own meals and baking your own baked goods to an already too-busy life. You must organize your whole life – not just your kitchen – to accomplish what you need to do. If you have family members who can help, take advantage of their offers of assistance. Organization will help you know what needs to be done and when, so you will be ready to give them specific helpful tasks.

Budget your time just as you budget a limited supply of money. We each have only 24 hours in a day and a finite number of days. Time is of greatest value if you are healthy enough to use it productively. Thus, anything you do to improve your health will pay off in increasing what you can accomplish overall.

Make a list of your tasks, priorities, and goals. You must decide which things are most important to you and then budget your time to reach these goals. Buy a day-timer and use it to record everything you need to do and when you need to do it. Look at it several times a day so that you do not forget anything. If your schedule gets too full, make some hard choices (based on your goals) and eliminate those activities that are least important. Do not over commit yourself to the extent that you start missing sleep; that is essential to good health also.

Although spending time cooking can be an adjustment if you have rarely cooked before, keep this in mind: in addition to being more expensive, dining in sit-down restaurants may take more time than you would spend cooking, eating, and cleaning up at home. If you feed yourself healthily at home and avoid reactions, you will be better able to do the other things you need to do. Eating at home will mean that you are saving money previously used to eat out. If your income is adequate, you may be able to spend some of that money to hire other things done; this will give you more time. Just *do it!* Put time for cooking in your schedule. Improve your health by cooking for yourself and staying on your diet. It's the best thing you can do for yourself and for your loved ones.

MENU PLANNING

Menu planning was discussed on pages 16 to 17 as it relates to saving money on grocery shopping. When you are planning a week's menus, along with reading the grocery ads and considering your budget, consult your day-timer and plan with the rest of your life in mind. If there is a day when you will be late getting home, plan a crock pot meal. Add a note to your schedule for the evening before your crock pot meal about readying the ingredients to throw in the crock pot the next morning. I even get my crock pot out and set it on the kitchen counter the night before.

On days when you will be home a short time (at least a half hour) before you want to have dinner, plan a quick-cooking entrée such as broiled meat, broiled, poached, or baked fish, or meat or poultry cooked quickly in a frying pan (see these recipes on pages 65 to 72), and serve it with quickly cooked vegetables and/or a salad. (See pages 117 to 123 for speedy salads).

On a day when you will be gone for just a few hours before dinner, especially if you have a time-bake feature on your oven, plan an oven meal. Prepare an oven entrée (see pages 74 to 79) or, more simply, get a roast to put in the oven along with an oven grain (see the recipe on page 80) or baked white or sweet potatoes and squash or a non-starchy vegetable. Some vegetables that we normally think of as quick-cooking, such as carrots and cabbage, are delicious when baked. (See the recipes on pages 82 to 85). If you have time, add an oven desert to the meal as well. (These recipes are on pages 154 and 155).

As you plan your weekly menus and grocery list, add notes to your day-timer about essential cooking tasks and when they need to be done.

If you regularly arrive home shortly before dinner, plan to cook on the week-end and stock your freezer with meals to eat during the week. Every weekend make a large batch or two of entrées or whole meals. Divide the leftovers into meal-sized portions and freeze them. After a few weekends of doing this, you will have quite an assortment of your favorite dishes frozen and will not have to eat the same thing two consecutive nights again. Each evening remove an entrée or meal from the freezer and put it in the refrigerator to thaw. The following day when you arrive home, all you have to do is heat the meal and possibly cook a vegetable and prepare a salad.

WASHING, PEELING AND CHOPPING

Preparation of fresh produce by washing, peeling and chopping is an area where you must find your own personal balance between saving time and saving money. If you have extra time (possibly due to the loss of a job) and can grow your own vegetables, purchase fruits and vegetables economically from a farmer or farmer's market, or are given free produce, you're not likely to fuss about the time you spend washing and preparing them! Enjoy the bounty of the fresh produce!

If you have apples to peel, especially with children to help you, consider investing in an old-fashioned crank-style apple peeler and corer made by Progressive International Corp. As I was preparing to revise this book, I got my old apple peeler out of the basement to see who made it and was amazed to find that these peelers are still available from the same company at the same address I used to order a replacement blade about fifteen years ago. This peeler can also be purchased from Amazon.com for $18 at the time of this writing. To use the peeler, push the set of three prongs into the core of an apple and turn the crank. In just a minute or two your apple will be skin-free (or nearly so) and cut into a long spiral of slices. Use a knife to remove any skin that the peeler missed and cut the cored, sliced apple in half lengthwise to produce half-slices that can be used in a pie.

However, if you are undet time pressure, you can save time by reducing your peeling and chopping of fruits and vegetables. Potatoes do not need to be peeled. Most of the nutrients are right under the skin, so if you scrub them thoroughly rather than peeling them, you will be getting better nutrition – and save time. I also scrub rather than peel the carrots I use in "Crock Pot Roast Dinner" (page 87) and other recipes where I use whole carrots. Pre-peeled mini carrots are great time savers, and many recipes in this book call for them.

Use pre-washed and prepared salad greens for salads. Frozen vegetables are pan-ready without washing or chopping. Although fresh-from-the-garden vegetables are the most nutritious, commercially produced vegetables are frozen soon after picking and retain more nutrients than vegetables that have been in transit or kept in the store's or your refrigerator for several days. Frozen vegetables are also often more economical.

Canned goods also can save you time on peeling and chopping. Use sugar-free canned beans to make "Three Bean Salad," page 120, quickly and economically. Use sugar-free water-packed canned apples to make apple crisp and other desserts quickly rather than peeling and slicing fresh apples. Canned apples are also less expensive than fresh if you must purchase apples at the grocery store when they are not on sale.

RECIPES AND MEASURING

It is common to see gluten-free baking recipes that call for a dozen or even twenty ingredients. The goal of these recipes is to produce the most normal baked goods possible, and this is done by using several flours together and small amounts of many stabilizing ingredients. A celiac friend assures me that these recipes do taste better, but there are trade-offs in terms of both time and allergies. If you bake with simpler recipes and do not eat the same things every day, you are less likely to develop an allergy to ingredients you use often. Furthermore, using recipes with fewer ingredients will save you time on measuring.

The ingredient lists for the recipes in this book are in most cases shorter than in some allergy and most gluten-free recipes books. Thus, it takes less time to measure the ingredients and make the recipe. In addition, when the ingredient list contains only the items which are absolutely necessary, those with food allergies are more likely to be able to use the recipe without leaving something out or trying to make a substitution. (See pages 59 to 60 for more about substitutions). Also, when an allergic reaction occurs after a meal and you only ate a few foods rather than a dozen or more, it is much easier to figure out which food was the problem.

BAKING

Those who must make most or all of their baked goods from scratch often feel they need to spend part of every day baking. The most efficient way to accomplish necessary baking without it taking over your life is to schedule a baking day every two weeks or once a month and do all of the baking at once. On that day you can make large batches and freeze most of what you bake. It is more convenient than getting out your measuring cups, baking pans and equipment for a small batch of muffins or crackers and cleaning up a baking mess every day or two.

However, if you eat mostly bread, and especially if you can have yeast, a baking day may not be necessary. With a bread machine (see pages 41 to 42) you can easily make a loaf of bread as often as you need it. If you rotate grains, when the rotation day for that type of bread ends, slice the rest of the loaf and freeze it. You can pull out the whole loaf or toast frozen slices of the bread the next time that rotation day comes around.

For more about baking, see pages 61 to 64.

CLEAN UP

Wash fewer dishes. Do anything you can to keep from getting another dish, pan or utensil dirty. Many of the recipes in this book cook multiple ingredients in one pan – first sauté the vegetables, then brown the meat in the same pan (or vice versa) and then put them all back together in that pan.

When you are measuring liquids for baking, measure all of the liquids together by adding them sequentially to the same 2-cup measuring cup. For instance, if you need ½ cup water, ¼ cup thawed apple juice concentrate, and ⅛ cup of oil, do this: Add water to the ½ cup line, add apple juice to the ¾ cup line, and then add oil to the ⅞ cup line. Stir them together right in the measuring cup and add them to the dry ingredients. That saves you having to wash an extra bowl used to combine the liquid ingredients.

Since most muffin tins must be washed by hand, line the cups with paper liners. This lessens the need for scrubbing to clean the muffin tin cups.

Although I do not cook in plastic myself (to avoid chemicals), if you have no chemical sensitivity, you might want to try the crock pot liners that you can purchase near the food storage bags in most grocery stores. They will save you having to scrub your crock pot after using it for a meal. Filling your crock pot with hot soapy water and letting it soak for a half hour or more before scrubbing also eases the cleaning task.

ENTERTAINING

In our busy modern lives, we usually have guests only a few times a year for such occasions as holidays or birthdays. Keep your menu simple when you have guests so you can enjoy their company. Having a meal in the oven or the crock pot (see the oven and crock pot meal chapters on pages 74 to 95) leaves you more time for visiting. If you must make something impressive, try the lasagne recipe on page 101 which can be prepared ahead. Use food as a tool to build relationships. Your friends will not remember how fancy the food you prepared was as long as they will remember how welcome they felt in your home.

MEDICAL TREATMENTS AS TIME-SAVERS

For those with food allergies, the treatment called low dose immunotherapy will use much of your time in the short run but can save you time in the long run by eliminating or lessening your sensitivities and improving your health. This allergy treatment, called Low Dose Allergens (LDA) in the United States or Enzyme Potentiated Desensitization (EPD) in Europe and Canada, is a type of allergy shots that are taken at two month intervals for about a year and then at longer intervals over several years time or possibly indefinitely. It is usually a treatment for the desperate because the dietary and environmental protocols that must be followed around the time of a shot can be an ordeal. However, if you are allergic to so many foods that you are near starvation or if you have chemical sensitivities, you may find the shots worth the effort. For more information see *The Ultimate Food Allergy Cookbook and Survival Guide* as described on the last pages of this book or consult the websites listed under "LDA and EPD" on page 222.

THE MOST IMPORTANT MONEY AND TIME-SAVER

The most important timesaving tip is this: Stay on your diet and faithfully follow whatever other instructions your doctor gives you. When you begin to feel better, it will seem as if you have twice (or several times) as much time. With improved energy levels and health you may be able to do things you have needed or wanted to do for a long while.

Know Your Ingredients

When you begin cooking for a celiac or food allergy diet you will encounter foods with which you are unfamiliar. They will taste different from what you are used to and will behave differently in cooking. Cooking with them will be much easier if you are prepared for these differences. This chapter is an introduction to some characteristics of the ingredients you will use on your diet.

Grains and Flours for
Celiac and Food Allergy Diets

The difference between gluten-free cooking and ordinary cooking is – obviously – that we use only gluten-free ingredients. On a gluten-free diet you will come to know gluten-free flours and other ingredients intimately and will realize that although gluten-free flours behave much differently than wheat (precisely because they lack gluten), they are delicious and produce wonderful foods.

The majority of the recipes in this book are gluten-free but for those whose allergies allow, some recipes contain gluten-containing grains. In addition, there are recipes that give the cook a choice of ingredients, so the recipe may or may not be gluten-free depending on which ingredients are used. The recipes that are always gluten-free are labeled:

Gluten-Free

Those that will be gluten-free with the correct ingredient choice are labeled:

Gluten-Free IF
made with millet

or the gluten-free ingredient choice. The abbreviation GF is used in recipe ingredient lists to indicate that a gluten-free variety or brand of the ingredient should be used to make the recipe gluten-free.

For both celiac and food allergy diets, see the index to the recipes by grain or grain alternative used on page 224 to easily find a recipe by the grain used. Because food allergy diets are not as uniform and well-defined as the celiac diet, those with food allergies will have to read recipes and decide which they can use based on their sensitivities. However, all of the recipes in this book are free of wheat and soy, most can be made without eggs, all but a few are dairy-free (and alternative milk is an option in most of those recipes), and "Cornbread" is the only corn-containing recipe.

GLUTEN-FREE TRUE GRAINS

Several of the flours used on a gluten-free diet are botanically classified as members of the grain family and therefore are true grains. All of these gluten-free grains are more crumbly than wheat in baked goods but have good flavor. The gluten-free true grains are:

CORN has a familiar and pleasant flavor. Cornmeal is widely available in grocery stores and adds an interesting texture to baked goods. Corn flour, which is similar to cornmeal but is ground to a smoother texture, is available at health food stores.

RICE is bland but pleasant tasting. Rice flour tends to be gritty in baked goods. Because rice is the main component of most commercially produced gluten-free baked goods, this book does not contain many rice recipes. You might as well let someone else cook it if you're going to eat rice! Rice and wild rice are closely related but are two different species. If you are allergic to rice, there is a chance that you may be able to eat wild rice.

TEFF is less bland than most of the gluten-free grains but is still delicious. It has been difficult to find in the past, but now Bob's Red Mill™ has made it readily available. If your health food store does not carry it, it is likely that they do carry some of Bob's other products and can easily get it in for you. Teff flour tends to be a little gritty but makes very nice baked products.

MILLET has excellent flavor. It is quite crumbly and tends to produce very dry baked goods no matter how much oil or pureed fruit you use in the recipe. Whole millet is delicious and is very easy to cook in the oven or on the stove top much as you would cook rice. (See the recipes on page 80 and 127). Millet and millet flour are usually available at health food stores. If your store doesn't carry them, you or your store can order them. For ordering information, see "Sources," page 210.

SORGHUM is sweet and delicious. It is also called **MILO** or **JOWAR**, and like millet, it tends to produce dry baked goods. It is used to make sorghum molasses and has traditionally been fed to cattle. Formerly very difficult to find, it now is produced by Authentic Foods™. (They also produce many other high quality organic gluten-free baking products). If your health food store does not carry sorghum flour, ask them to get it in for you. For ordering information, see "Sources," page 210.

OATS have a delicious familiar flavor. Recently some doctors have begun to allow oats on gluten-free diets. Since oats do contain a low level of gluten-like proteins, it is possible that not all celiacs will tolerate them. Oats often produce heavy baked goods, and an occasional batch of oat flour may yield gummy products. However, they are still edible and satisfying.

NON-GRAINS

The non-grains are not botanically related to wheat and do not contain gluten. Many of them are the seeds of plants so they are very nutritious and high in protein. In the recipes in this book, the seed flours are often used with small quantities of a starch to help them stick together. The non-grains include:

AMARANTH is in the same botanical order as quinoa, although it is not in the same food family. Because it is not a grain, it is a welcome dietary addition for those allergic to all grains. It makes very tasty baked goods. Purchase it at a store that refrigerates its flour and refrigerate or freeze it at home since it may develop a strong flavor if stored too long at room temperature. An occasional batch of amaranth flour will yield gummy pancakes or bread, but the recipes included in this book (crackers, muffins, cookies) rarely have this problem.

QUINOA boasts a high content of high-quality protein. Due to its amino acid balance, it is one of the best protein sources among plant foods. For this reason, it is very satisfying to eat; quinoa baked goods really stick with you. Those allergic to all grains will find quinoa a welcome dietary staple. It has a distinctive taste so goes well with other strongly flavored ingredients such as cinnamon, sesame seeds and carob. Quinoa flour is excellent in baked goods of all kinds and makes good yeast bread. Whole grain quinoa has a natural soapy coating on it, so before you cook it, put it in a strainer and rinse it under running water until the water is no longer sudsy. This coating protects the plant from insects. Quinoa is in the same food family as spinach, beets, and Swiss chard.

BUCKWHEAT is a very versatile non-grain flour. It is excellent in waffles and pancakes, and a chocolate-eating celiac friend raves about "Chocolate Brownies," page 156, made with buckwheat flour. In a few recipes (such crackers and muffins, which are not included in this book) it can have a strong flavor. It is in the same food family as rhubarb.

BEAN FLOURS such as GARBANZO, GARFAVA, and FAVA FLOUR are also high protein additions to the gluten-free diet. They do not stick together well and must be used with larger quantities of other flours or starches.

CAROB POWDER is also a bean flour since carob beans are in the legume family. It is usually used as a chocolate substitute rather than as the main ingredient of baked goods. Carob flour or powder is naturally sweet, so it does not require as much additional sweetener in recipes as chocolate does. It tends to form hard lumps upon standing, so you may need to press it through a wire mesh strainer with the back of a spoon before using it. Carob bean gum (also called locust bean gum) is derived from the bean of the carob plant and is used in many commercially prepared foods. Carob chips are a welcome addition to cookies for those who are allergic to chocolate.

There are several white, highly refined starches that are commonly used in gluten-free cooking. They include **ARROWROOT, TAPIOCA FLOUR/STARCH, WATER CHESTNUT STARCH, CORNSTARCH,** and **BEAN STARCH.** These starches serve as binders in gluten-free baking and can also be used as thickeners for sauces and gravies. Arrowroot and tapioca starch can be substituted for each other in baking in equal quantities. Tapioca and cassava are made from the tuber of the same plant; tapioca is just more highly refined.

POTATO FLOUR and **POTATO STARCH** (also called potato starch flour) also may be used in gluten-free cooking. They are not the same thing, however, and cannot be used interchangeably. Potato flour is made from whole potatoes and retains the nutritional value of potatoes including considerable protein. In baking, it must be used with eggs (usually it is folded into beaten egg whites) or the baked product may end up like mashed potatoes on the inside. Potato starch is a highly refined starch, much like the starches in the preceding paragraph, except that it attracts and holds moisture, or is hygroscopic. Both of these ingredients must be used in small amounts in most recipes or their hygroscopic nature may cause a gooey texture in the final product.

Exotic flours such as **CHESTNUT FLOUR, CASSAVA MEAL or FLOUR,** and **TUBER FLOURS** are useful for individuals sensitive to all grains. Cassava meal can be used for breading meat and fish and for crackers and is not too expensive. Cassava flour (also called manioc or mandioca) is more expensive and is the flour contained in the gluten-free Chebe™ bread mixes you may find in your health food store. Chestnut flour and flours made from a variety of unusual tubers may be needed by those with extremely extensive food allergies but they are expensive. For recipes made with these flours, see *The Ultimate Food Allergy Cookbook and Survival Guide* which is described on the last pages of this book.

GLUTEN-CONTAINING GRAINS FOR ALLERGY DIETS

In addition to the gluten-free grains and flours discussed on the preceding pages, some people who are allergic to wheat but are not sensitive to gluten can eat the following grains:

BARLEY is a very pleasant tasting gluten-containing grain in the same tribe of the grain family as rye, spelt, kamut, and wheat. Baked goods made with barley flour have a very pleasant flavor but tend to be crumbly.

KAMUT is a golden yellow grain with very good flavor. Kamut is very closely related to wheat in its biological classification, being in the same genus but a different species. However, some people who are allergic to wheat can eat kamut without reacting. Kamut seems to be tolerated by fewer wheat-sensitive individuals than spelt however. Kamut makes good yeast breads and very tasty non-yeast baked goods, although they are likely to be dense.

RYE is a very versatile, tasty grain. It contains a fair amount of gluten and behaves much like whole wheat flour in baking. It has a slightly stronger flavor than some of the other grains but is delicious in breads. Rye is in the same tribe of the grain family as barley, spelt, kamut, and wheat.

SPELT is probably the most versatile non-wheat grain. Spelt is very closely related to wheat in its biological classification, being *Triticum spelta* while wheat is *Triticum aestivum*. (See "The Spelt-Wheat Debate" on pages 219 to 220 for more about this). In spite of the close relationship, spelt is tolerated by many wheat-sensitive individuals. Muffins and cakes made with spelt flour tend to be a little drier than those made with other grains, and so the recipes may contain more oil. Spelt makes excellent yeast bread because it is as high in gluten as wheat although its gluten is more soluble. You may purchase sifted or white spelt flour which has had the bran sifted out but is not processed in any other way. Baked goods made with white spelt often are nearly indistinguishable from normal baked goods. Therefore, if you can eat spelt, have it on the days that you have guests. They may not be able to tell that your white spelt dessert or bread is even different.

All of the spelt recipes in this book were developed using Purity Foods™ flour. Purity Foods mills its flour from a European strain of spelt that is higher in protein than most spelt flours. In the years since I first began baking with spelt, several other companies have also begun to produce spelt flour. These other flours do not work well in the recipes in this book and are unsuitable for yeast breads. If you use them in non-yeast baked goods, you will have to add more flour than the recipes call for and expect less satisfactory results. It is worth the effort to get Purity Foods flour. Many health food stores carry it (if yours doesn't, ask them to get it in) or see "Sources of Special Foods," page 210, for ordering information.

Leavenings and Binders

Leavenings are the ingredients that make baked products rise. They include baking powder, baking soda combined with an acid ingredient, and yeast. Binders help the leavenings work by trapping the gas the leavenings produce. They are not needed when you bake with wheat because the gluten in wheat flour forms sheets that trap the gas. Binders include eggs, starches (discussed on page 53), and fibers such as guar gum and xanthum gum.

BAKING POWDER is a combination of acid and basic components that, when moistened, produces gas to make baked goods rise in baking. Some brands of baking powder contain aluminum which should probably be avoided for best health. Bob's Red Mill™ produces a good aluminum-free baking powder which is sold in large economical bags. I store Bob's™ baking powder in small jars to keep it dry and potent until I finish using the whole bag. Most commercial baking powder contains cornstarch. If you are sensitive to corn, use Featherweight™ baking powder which contains potato starch instead of cornstarch and is also sodium-free. Baking powder reacts slowly after contact with liquids and leavens a little less rapidly than baking soda plus vitamin C powder so is used in some of the recipes in this book where that is needed.

BAKING SODA is pure sodium bicarbonate and is almost universally tolerated by people with severe food allergies. For those on rotation diets, it is usually allowed every day of the rotation cycle. It must be used in conjunction with an acid ingredient to make baked goods rise. The acid ingredients commonly used in standard cooking include buttermilk, lemon juice or other fruit juices, and cream of tartar. For the very allergic, unbuffered vitamin C powder is the best way to provide the acid component of the leavening process. (Buffered vitamin C, however, will not provide the acid needed for leavening). Hypoallergenic vitamin C is very pure and is also usually allowed on every day of the rotation diet. See "Sources," page 211, for cassava-source vitamin C.

Some of the recipes in this book and most of the recipes in *The Ultimate Food Allergy Cookbook and Survival Guide* and *Allergy Cooking with Ease* contain a built-in baking powder made of baking soda and unbuffered vitamin C powder.

BAKER'S YEAST is what makes commercial bread rise and is available in many forms. Active dry yeast is yeast that has been freeze-dried to retain its activity. An expiration date is usually stamped on the package and the yeast should be good until that date if you store it in the refrigerator after opening it. Active dry yeast is available in ¼ ounce (2¼ teaspoon) packets or 4 ounce jars in most grocery stores. In addition, you can purchase it in one pound bags and store the yeast in your freezer. Do not thaw and refreeze this yeast; instead occasionally take out a small amount to use within a few weeks and keep it in a jar in the refrigerator. Leave the remainder of the yeast frozen. Red Star™ active dry yeast is free of gluten and preservatives and works well in bread machines. Instant or quick-rise yeasts such as SAF™ leaven bread more rapidly than active dry yeast so they are useful for making bread more quickly. These fast types of yeast are not recommended for gluten-free bread because its structure is more fragile. If quick-rise yeast is used, the bread may over-rise and then collapse during baking.

EGGS and **FRUIT PUREES** are binders that also are used in normal baking. These ingredients hold your baked goods together and add nutritional value and flavor.

GUAR GUM and **XANTHUM GUM** are two types of soluble fiber used as binders in gluten-free baking. They both can be fairly allergenic, so I use them only in yeast breads where they are actually essential. If you have problems with one of them, you can substitute the other in the same amount in recipes. Guar gum is made from a legume. Xanthum gum is derived from a type of bacteria, *Xanthomonas compestris,* which may be grown on a corn-based medium.

Sweeteners

Most of the recipes in this book are sweetened with liquid fruit sweeteners rather than sugar. Fruit sweeteners contain fructose, a simple sugar which can be directly absorbed without any digestion and does not cause wide swings in blood sugar levels as refined sugar (sucrose) does. Although honey, molasses, and date sugar may contribute more to blood sugar problems, they are not highly refined and contain many minerals and other nutrients.

LIQUID FRUIT SWEETENERS make delicious and healthy baked goods. The least concentrated of these are pureed fruits and fruit juice followed by fruit juice concentrates. Apple juice concentrate is used in many of the recipes in this book. I routinely keep a can of apple juice concentrate in my refrigerator so I'm always ready to bake. More concentrated liquid fruit sweeteners include Fruit Sweet™ which is a blend of pear and pineapple juice concentrates, Pear Sweet™ and Grape Sweet™. Using these sweeteners, you can make desserts so similar to sugar-containing desserts that no one will know they do not contain sugar. They are used in only a few recipes in this book because many health food stores do not carry them, but they can be ordered easily and make such good desserts that they are very much worth ordering. See "Sources," page 214 for information about ordering these sweeteners.

DATE SUGAR is ground dried dates. It is a concentrated sweetener which is very useful in desserts where more sweetness is desired. It also helps keep your baked goods moist. It is the only dry sweetener routinely used in this book.

HONEY and **MOLASSES** are less refined sweeteners that add moistness and flavor to baked goods. Honey is used in some recipes in this book where more sweetness is desired than can be achieved with fruit juice concentrates. Molasses is used in the gingerbread recipe. Although they are potent sweeteners which may have more effect on blood sugar levels than fruit sweeteners, unlike white sugar, they have not been stripped of their minerals and other nutrients.

AGAVE is a relatively new liquid sweetener. This low glycemic index unrefined sweetener comes from a plant in the yucca family and has much less effect on blood sugar levels than other caloric sweeteners. Since it is sweeter than sugar it can be used in smaller amounts, thus saving calories. It is about 90% fructose and 10% glucose. Agave is a wonderful sweetener for coffee or tea. In baking it seems stickier than other sweeteners, so if you use it to make cookies, be sure to line your baking sheets with parchment paper for easy removal of the cookies

This new natural sweetener will be featured in an upcoming dessert cookbook for allergy and celiac diets. Visit the book page of my website (www.food-allergy. org/books.html) any time after the summer of 2009 for more information.

RICE SYRUP is another sweetener which may be allowed on gluten-free diets if it is made without barley or other grains. However, since most rice syrup is not gluten-free, it is not used in the recipes in this book. It is less sweet than fruit sweeteners. Baked products made with rice syrup do not brown as much as those made with other sweeteners.

SUGAR is an ingredient which I normally avoid using. It has been stripped of the nutrients naturally present in sugar cane or sugar beets and is so highly refined that it can have a profound effect on blood sugar levels and intestinal flora. When I heard Dr. William Crook speak to a group of medical professionals years ago, he was asked many questions about the best diet for those with candidiasis. He said there was only one absolute prohibition, and that was sugar. In his experience he had found that even if patients took potent systemic anti-fungal medications, if they continued to eat sugar, their intestinal *Candida* could not be controlled. Sugar also "feeds" unfriendly intestinal bacteria and parasites. For these reasons, sugar can potentially make food allergies worse from the effect it has on intestinal flora and thus on intestinal permeability.

However, sugar is used in one recipe in this book – the chocolate brownie recipe – because celiac friends love these brownies and there are no longer non-sucrose dry sweeteners on the market that give these brownies a normal taste and texture. I used to make sugar-free chocolate brownies using Fruit Source™ but the company that made that product has vanished. If you make these brownies, please save them and other sugar-containing goodies for special occasions rather than eating them routinely even if you do not have *Candida* or other problems with intestinal flora. For more information about intestinal health and food allergies, see *The Ultimate Food Allergy Cookbook and Survival Guide* which is described on the last pages of this book.

Thickeners

Most of the thickeners used in the recipes in this book require cooking. They include white, highly refined starches such as **ARROWROOT, TAPIOCA FLOUR/STARCH,** and **CORNSTARCH.** When cooked with water, these thickeners form a nearly-clear liquid. They are great for making sauces and gravies, although the gravies look different (less opaque) than when thickened with flour. Sauces thickened with tapioca tend to be a little more ropy than those thickened with arrowroot or cornstarch, and you may need slightly more tapioca than arrowroot or cornstarch to produce the same amount of thickening.

Instant thickeners such as **QUICKTHICK**™ and **THICKENUP**™ are thickeners that do not require cooking. QuickThick™ formerly was available in a nearby cooking specialty store but is no longer carried there. It is slightly better than ThickenUp™ for keeping the oil from separating in salad dressings. Since Quick-Thick™ and ThickenUp™ are a type of corn starch, they cannot be used by people with corn allergy. The new canister of ThickenUp™ which I recently purchased is labeled as both gluten- and lactose-free. Both thickeners are available in pharmacies or on the Internet as an aid for stroke victims and others who have trouble swallowing thin liquids.

Main Dish Ingredients to Be Careful About

The ingredients listed below are tasty to use in main dishes and are used in a few recipes in this book, but grocery store brands can be troublesome to those with food allergies or gluten intolerance because of what may be added to them. However, if you shop carefully and read labels, you should be able to find brands that you can use if you have celiac disease or your allergies are not too extensive. When in doubt, use the option (given in the recipes in this book) of water instead of broth or wine. In addition, see the information on pages 28 to 29 about added ingredients to watch for in any canned vegetables or tomato products which you may use in main dishes.

BROTHS bought at a grocery store almost always contain monosodium glutamate (MSG) which is problematic for celiacs, people who are allergic to wheat, and many normal people as well. When I recently read several cans of broth at the grocery store, I discovered that in addition to MSG, they also contained a list of ingredients including all the major food allergens: hydrolyzed wheat gluten, autolyzed yeast extract, dextrose, high fructose corn syrup, hydrolyzed soy protein, hydrolyzed corn protein, soy lecithin, caramel color, maltodextrin, sugar, cane juice solids (in a "natural" broth), yeast extract, rice extract, corn syrup solids, and dry whey. In addition, many of them contained two ingredients I did not recognize – disodium inosinate and disodium guanylate. I learned that these are two flavor enhancers that amplify the effect of MSG!

But take heart, you do not have to start with a chicken and water to have broth. There are several brands carried in health food stores that have no such additives. See "Using Commercially Prepared Foods," pages 202 to 204 for more information about these broths.

WINE can tenderize meat and add a delicious flavor to main dishes. However, wines are out for people allergic to yeast and sometimes also are treated with sulfites or may be clarified with eggs. Call the winery to double check the wine you wish to drink or use in cooking. Your chances of being able to use it are better if you choose an organic wine such as Bonterra. (See "Special Diet Resources," page 208). When in doubt, anyone suffering from food allergies should use the water option in this book's recipes calling for wine.

Ingredient Substitutions

When you bake for a gluten-free or food allergy diet, you will need to purchase many new ingredients. If you have forgotten to buy one of them, you may wonder if you can substitute something else for that new ingredient you do not have on hand! Substitutions are tricky in gluten-free and allergy baking. The recipes in this book should work as written (although an unusual batch of flour from a health food store bulk bin can upset any recipe). If you substitute, there are no guarantees.

People call me and say, "I've got your recipe made with quinoa flour and I want to make it with oat flour. How can I do this?" I usually can't give them a definite answer, although I try to make suggestions that may or may not work. In my experience, there is no rule or conversion factor for substitutions between any two types of flour that will work predictably in all types of recipes. The flour conversion tables you may have seen are based on how much liquid each type of flour absorbs but do not account for other properties of the flour.

The bottom line on flour substitutions is this: be prepared to tweak a recipe made with a substitute flour several times before it is right, and realize that there are some recipes in which a desired substitution will not work. If there is not a recipe for something you want in this book, see *The Ultimate Food Allergy Cookbook and Survival Guide* as described on the last pages of this book. Because that book is designed to be the ultimate help for people whose diets may be extremely limited, I attempted to make each type of flour into as many types of recipes as possible and only omitted a certain recipe if it really was not possible to make. For example, since buckwheat can be bitter in crackers and muffins, these recipes were not included in this book. However, since there are severely allergic people who can eat only one or two grain alternatives, recipes for buckwheat crackers and muffins are in *The Ultimate Food Allergy Cookbook and Survival Guide.*

Unlike wheat flour, milk is an ingredient where substitutions in normal recipes usually work. In most recipes, you can replace the milk with an equal amount of water. Sometimes you can replace milk with fruit juice, but the acidity of the juice can affect the leavening process and result in a collapse of your baked product. Gluten-free yeast breads, in which the protein content contributed by the milk helps strengthen the structure of the bread, can be an exception to the rule that water can be substituted for milk.

In allergy baking, eggs usually can be replaced with an equal volume of water if the recipe is not depending on the egg for structure. However, in a recipe made with a gluten-free or low gluten flour, the egg sometimes is serving to replace part of the structure normally provided by gluten. Thus, replacing the egg with water may lead to a collapse.

Home ground flour also may behave differently from commercially ground flour, and it can vary from batch to batch of grain. If you use either very finely milled flour or coarsely milled or blender-ground flour, you will have to change the amount of liquid used in the recipe. Unless you are willing to experiment with each new batch of grain when you grind your own flour, it is best to purchase flour from a reliable commercial source.

If you are pressed for time, my advice about substitutions is don't try it unless it is one of the usually-works situations mentioned above. In the long run, you will waste less time and money if you run to the store for the missing ingredient or find and use a recipe written for the food you want to make using the grain you want to use and ingredients that you tolerate.

Baking with Ease

Baking can be the bugaboo of celiac and food allergy diets. Especially for those on rotation diets, it can seem that every day brings another batch (or batches) of muffins, crackers, or bread to be made. How can we bake successfully in a limited amount of time? This chapter will give you techniques to bring baking under control and make it less intrusive on your life.

When we have to do something that we are not confident or enthusiastic about, the first step towards dealing with it better may be to ask and answer the question "Why?" Thinking about the reasons for baking may help. The basic reason for baking for your special diet is to have tasty grain-based foods that are economical, safe for your diet, and that you know you can eat without consequences. A gluten-free or food allergy diet is expensive is because commercially-made muffins, breads and crackers are expensive. It follows that the best way to save money on your diet is to bake for yourself. You cannot just quit eating well; restricting your diet for economic reasons is counterproductive to optimal health. Complex carbohydrates are an important part of a healthy diet. They provide energy, fiber, and essential nutrients. If our diets consist only of protein foods, fruits and vegetables, we may feel unsatisfied, like something is missing, and indeed, we maybe be missing essential nutrients. Bread is truly the staff of life. If you are on a rotation diet, even if you can afford to buy any pre-made food available, the variety is limited. You may need homemade foods for some days of the diet. Celiacs with any tendency toward allergy are also wise not to eat rice every day and to vary their grains by making their own baked products.

An additional reason to bake at home is that freshly made breads and other baked goods are delicious. They satisfy the soul as well as the body and simply taste better than something that has been sitting in a health food store freezer for days or weeks. Nothing compares to the smell of freshly baked bread, muffins, or cookies.

Baking is not difficult, but there are a few basic facts that you should know to insure good results. Since this is information may be a review for many readers, you can skim ahead a few pages to the time-saving tips if you have heard it already.

Here is a summary of baking basics: The first thing to do is to purchase the correct ingredients. High quality flour that is consistent from bag to bag will save you money, time and trouble in the long run. Authentic Foods™, Arrowhead Mills™ and Bob's Red Mill™ are brands that I use and recommend for most types of alternative flour. If you are can tolerate spelt, always use Purity Food™ brand flour. I have encountered more variability in spelt flour than in other types of flour, and it is not worth it to save a few pennies by purchasing an unknown brand from a health food store bulk bin if you might end up with bread that no one wants to eat. If you use other brands of spelt flour for non-yeast baked goods, you will have to add more flour than the recipes call for and expect less satisfactory results. If you use them for yeast bread, don't be surprised by collapsed loaves.

Be careful about what you purchase for other ingredients also. If you are leavening your baked goods with baking soda plus vitamin C, be sure that the vitamin C powder or crystals that you use are unbuffered. If you are allergic to corn, also make sure they are corn-free. (See "Sources," page 211, for information about ordering cassava-source unbuffered vitamin C). Your baking powder should be gluten-free and/or corn-free to fit your sensitivities. When you purchase baking mixes, be sure to read the label carefully every time because the ingredients may have changed.

The second baking basic is measuring ingredients accurately. Use the right measuring cups for the ingredient you are measuring – nested sets for flour and other solids ingredients and glass or plastic cups with markings for liquids. To measure flour, stir the flour to loosen it. Using a large spoon, lightly spoon the flour into the cup. Level it off with a straight edged knife or spatula. If you are measuring an amount of flour that you do not have a measuring cup for such as ⅝ cup, use the table of measurements on page 223 to determine how to measure it. In this case it is by using a ½ cup plus ⅛ cup.

To measure liquids, fill the cup with liquid until the meniscus (the bottom of the curve of the liquid) lines up with the line on the cup that is the amount you want to measure. Get down on your knees so you can read the cup at eye level as it sits on your counter. If your recipe calls for several liquids, you can save yourself time on washing an extra bowl by measuring them all in the same measuring cup and mixing them there before adding them to the dry ingredients. See page 48 for an example of how to do this.

To measure small amounts of flour, starch, salt, baking powder, spices, and other dry ingredients with measuring spoons, dip the spoon into the container, stir up the ingredient to loosen it, and fill the spoon generously. Pull it out and level it off with a straight edged knife or spatula, or level spices using the straight edge of the hole in the spice container. To measure small amounts of liquids, pour the liquid into the measuring spoon until it is level with the top of the spoon. Do not let it bead up over the top of the spoon.

The third baking technique that is crucial to success is proper mixing. Because the types of flour used in special diet baking produce a more fragile structure which must trap the gas produced by the leavening, how you mix non-yeast baked goods and how quickly you get them into the oven is very important. Before you begin baking, preheat your oven. Prepare the baking pans ahead of time; oil and flour them with the same oil and flour used in the recipe. Mix the dry ingredients together in a large bowl and the liquid ingredients together in your measuring cup or another bowl. Working quickly, stir the liquid ingredients into the dry ingredients until they are **just mixed.** It is critical that you do not mix for too long or the leavening will produce most of its gas in the mixing bowl rather than in the baking pan in the oven. Only stir until the dry ingredients are barely moistened; a few floury spots in your batter or dough are all right. As soon as you have mixed just enough, quickly put the batter or dough into the prepared baking pans and pop them into the preheated oven.

To test quick breads, muffins, and cakes for doneness, insert a toothpick into the center of the pan. If it comes out dry, it is time to remove the pan from the oven. Most baked goods should be removed from the pan immediately after you take them from the oven, but some fragile cakes and cookies benefit from cooling in the pan for about 10 minutes. The recipe will tell you when to do this. Allow your baked goods to cool on a cooling rack before you slice them or store them in a bag. While plastic bags and containers are great for storing most baked goods, crackers will stay crisp if you store them in a metal tin.

TIME-SAVING TECHNIQUES FOR BAKING

Some celiac readers probably have several *Gluten-Free Gourmet* cookbooks and have favorite baking recipes that use Bette Hagman's gluten-free flour mixes. One time-saving tip for using her recipes is to make up the flour mixes in batches large enough to last you for six months or more and store them in a cool place or freeze them. This will save you time on mixing the flour before you bake. If you have more money than time, Authentic Foods™ produces some of her flour mixes, so you can purchase some of them pre-mixed. See "Special Diet Resources," page 197, for contact and ordering information for Authentic Foods.

For people with food allergies, the ratios of ingredients in recipes are less constant from one food to another than in recipes for celiacs. For instance, although I almost always pair amaranth flour with arrowroot in baking, the proportions vary from recipe to recipe. So rather than making flour mixes, you might make baking mixes to save time. For example, when you are making amaranth muffins, get out a few plastic bags in addition to your mixing bowl. Measure the one-batch amount of amaranth flour, arrowroot, baking soda, and vitamin C (and optional cloves if you prefer them in your muffins) into each bag as well as into the bowl. Label each bag with the recipe, name of the book the recipe came from, page number, and date. If you have included optional ingredients in the bags and sometimes make this recipe without the optional ingredients, you may wish to write that on the bag also. Store the bags in a cool place. The next time you want to make amaranth muffins, all you will have to do is measure and add the liquid ingredients.

If you have enough freezer space, the best way to prevent baking from taking up too much of your life is to have a baking day every few weeks and bake large batches of everything you will need in the near future on that day. You will only have to get out your mixing bowls, measuring cups, ingredients, and baking pans once, and you will have a baking mess in your kitchen to clean up on only one day rather than on several. At the end of the day, freeze most of what you made and it will be ready to pull out of the freezer when you want to eat it. If you slice bread before freezing it, you do not need to take it out to thaw before you are going to eat it. Just pull out individual frozen slices from the freezer and toast them in a toaster oven. (Alternative breads are often too fragile for pop-up toasters). Those on a rotation diet should always use the same flour, oil, and sweetener together. If your rotation is consistent in this way, frozen baked goods can be eaten the next time that rotation day arrives.

With a small freezer, you can still have baking days to reduce the need to spend time baking often. On your baking day, make small batches of your special foods and also make bags of baking mixes as described on the previous page at the same time. Freeze your small batches or what is uneaten from them at the end of the day. When you finish eating a small batch you have in the freezer, you will save time on making its replacement by starting with a baking mix rather than with each separate dry ingredient.

A final very nutritious solution for reducing the amount of baking required by your diet is to do less baking and eat cooked whole grains instead of baked goods. This type of diet – and the amount of work involved – is likely to be welcomed by an adult who is not terribly fussy about what he or she eats, but only is interested in nutrition. It is also likely to be usable with a child too young to know or care about what the other children are eating. Whole grains can be cooked on the stove top or in the oven. (These recipes are on pages 80 and 126). If you have space in your freezer and want to save work, cook large batches of the grains you can eat and freeze them in small portions for future use.

Dinner in a Jiffy

Dinner preparation won't take long if you choose foods that cook quickly. This chapter contains recipes for quick-cooking entrées that will let you have table-ready food in a half hour or less. Serve the entrées with a vegetable (quickly cooked on the stove top or in the microwave), a salad, and fresh fruit for dessert and – voila! – a delicious, nutritious meal in record time.

Some of the quick meal cookbooks I studied as I was preparing to write this book included recipes for undercooked meat, raw fish, and other foods that might be potential health hazards if you consider their microbiology. Since I believe in thoroughly cooking all animal foods for safety, that is how the dishes in this book are cooked. This chapter also incorporates a few food safety lessons into the recipes.

These recipes include two tasty, quick-baking, not-plain fish dishes and creative ways to prepare thin pieces of turkey, chicken, or beef in a frying pan with wine and a gluten-free starch based sauce. The recipes also include very basic instructions on how to broil steaks, hamburgers, or lamb chops as well as how to poach, broil or bake fish, how to cook pasta, and even a quick chili recipe. If you have been cooking for years, please do not take offence at these basic recipes. People often call me who just found out they have to be on a celiac or allergy diet and their meal preparation experience has been limited to microwaving frozen entrées. One person told me, "I'm the queen of fast food." So if you're a cook rather than a fast food fan, just skip over the basic recipes on pages 70 to 73 and move on to the more creative recipes in the next chapter.

Basil Roughy

`Gluten-Free`

This dish is delicious, tender, and will be on the table in nearly no time.

1 pound orange roughy fillets
1½ to 2 tablespoons oil or melted butter
1 tablespoon lemon juice OR ¼ teaspoon unbuffered vitamin C powder
    plus 1 tablespoon water (optional)
⅛ teaspoon salt, or to taste
Dash of paprika (optional)
½ teaspoon dry sweet basil

If you are using the vitamin C, mix it with the water in a corner of a 9-inch by 13-inch glass baking dish until it is dissolved. Combine the oil or melted butter with the vitamin C solution or lemon juice in the baking dish. Put the fillets into the dish and turn them over so they are coated with the oil mixture on both sides. Sprinkle them with the salt, paprika, and basil. Bake at 350°F for about 15 minutes, or until the fish flakes easily with a fork. Makes 2 to 4 servings.

Ann Fisk's Baked Fish

Gluten-Free

1 pound fillets of orange roughy, tilapia, or other mild-flavored fish of
    your choice
2 to 4 teaspoons of olive oil or other oil, butter, or ghee
Dash of paprika (optional)
Salt and pepper to taste

Preheat your oven to 400°F. Lay the fish in a single layer in a glass baking dish. If the fillets have skin, lay them skin side down. Dot the fish with the butter or ghee or drizzle it with the oil. To give the fish an appealing color, sprinkle it with paprika. Put it into the oven and bake it until it is opaque throughout and flakes easily with a fork. The cooking time will be about 5 to 10 minutes warm-up time plus 10 minutes per inch of thickness of the fish. Sprinkle the fish with salt and pepper if desired. Serve immediately. Makes 3 to 4 servings.

Sweet salmon variation: Use salmon and drizzle it before baking with 2 tablespoons of orange juice and 2 teaspoons of honey in addition to the oil.

Turkey Piccata

Gluten-Free

A little wine adds a lot of class to the next three quick-cooking recipes.

1 to 1¼ pounds of sliced turkey breast
2 tablespoons oil, preferably olive oil
3 tablespoons tapioca starch, arrowroot, or cornstarch
¼ to ½ teaspoon salt
Dash of pepper
2 tablespoons lemon juice
½ cup white wine or water

Mix the starch, salt, and pepper together in a plate or on a piece of waxed paper. Dip the turkey slices into the mixture so both sides are coated. While you are dipping the turkey, heat the oil in a large* frying pan (large enough to hold all the slices in a single layer) over medium to medium-high heat for a minute or so. Add the turkey breast slices to the pan and cook them for about 3 minutes on one side until they are beginning to brown. Turn them over and brown them on the other side also for about 3 minutes. Add the lemon juice and wine to the pan. Reduce the heat and simmer uncovered for 3 to 5 minutes until the liquid begins to thicken. Turn the turkey slices. Cover the pan with a lid and simmer for another 5 minutes. Check the pan after 2 to 3 minutes and add more water or wine if the liquid is drying out. If necessary, at the end of the cooking time remove the lid and simmer until the liquid is very thick like a glaze covering the turkey. Serve immediately. Makes 3 to 4 servings.

Note: If you are making this dinner for one or two people and do not have a large frying pan, halve the amounts of all the ingredients and cook it in a smaller pan.

Chicken Marsala

Gluten-Free

2 whole skinless boned chicken breasts (about 2 pounds)
1½ to 2 tablespoon olive oil or other oil
3 to 4 tablespoons tapioca starch, arrowroot, or cornstarch
Dash of salt
Dash of pepper
1 4-ounce (dry weight) can of mushrooms, not drained (7 ounces
    total weight)*
½ cup GF Marsala wine, grape juice, or water*

Pound the chicken breasts with a meat tenderizer until they are thin. Mix the starch, salt and pepper together in a plate or on a piece of waxed paper. Dip the chicken into the mixture so both sides are coated. While you are preparing the chicken, heat the oil in a large* frying pan (large enough to hold all the chicken in a single layer) over medium to medium-high heat for a minute or so. Add the chicken pieces to the pan and cook them for about 3 minutes on one side until they are beginning to brown. Turn them over and brown them on the other side also for about 3 minutes. Add the mushrooms with their juice and the Marsala, juice or water to the pan. Cover the pan and bring the liquid to a boil. Reduce the heat and simmer for 15 minutes. Turn the pieces of chicken over half-way through the simmering time so both sides absorb the sauce. As the simmering time nears its end, check the pan and add more water or wine if the liquid is drying out. If the sauce does not thicken quickly enough, at the end of 15 minutes remove the lid from the pan and simmer another few minutes until the sauce is thick. Serve immediately. Makes 4 servings.

*Notes: If you are allergic to yeast and wish to make this recipe, omit the mushrooms and use ¾ cup of juice or water instead of the wine.

If you are making this dinner for one or two people and do not have a large frying pan, halve the amounts of all the ingredients and cook it in a smaller pan.

Quick Stroganoff

Gluten-Free IF
noodles are GF

1 to 1½ pounds of beef for stir-fry or fairly tender steak

1 8- to 13-ounce (dry weight) can mushrooms, drained, or ¾ pound
 fresh mushrooms, sliced (optional)

1 small onion, chopped, or 3 to 4 tablespoons dry chopped onions
 (optional)

1½ to 2 tablespoons oil (Use the larger amount if more meat is used).

1 teaspoon salt, only if the beef broth is not used

2 tablespoons tapioca starch, arrowroot, or cornstarch

1 to 1¼ cups GF red wine, GF beef broth, or water (Use the larger
 amount if more meat is used).

4 cups cooked noodles such as rice noodles, quinoa noodles, or other
 noodles acceptable on your diet

If you are using the fresh vegetables, sauté them in the oil in a frying pan until they are tender. While the vegetables are cooking, prepare the steak by cutting it into thin strips about 2 inches long. Also begin cooking the noodles while you wait. (Directions for cooking pasta are on page 73). When the vegetables are tender, remove them from the pan. If there is no oil left, add an additional tablespoon of oil to the pan and proceed as in the second paragraph below.

If you are not using the fresh vegetables, add the oil to a frying pan. Prepare the steak as above. (Using pre-cut stir-fry meat will save you some time on this step).

Cook the meat over medium-high heat in the oil for 5 to 7 minutes or until it is brown on all sides. Mix together the starch and the wine, broth, or water and add them to the meat. Add the cooked vegetables, canned mushrooms, or dry onions to the pan. Add the salt if you did not use the broth. Bring the pan to a boil over medium-high heat and cook for a few minutes until the sauce has thickened. Serve over hot cooked noodles. Makes 4 servings

Game Stroganoff variation: Use any red game meat steak instead of beef. After browning the meat, add 1½ cups of water to the pan and simmer the meat for 45 minutes. Proceed with the recipe as above except use only ¾ cup of wine, broth or additional water to mix with the starch.

Broiled Beef or Lamb Steak or Chops

Gluten-Free

The rules of food safety for cooking solid cuts of meat such as beef or lamb steaks, chops, and roasts differ from the rules for cooking ground meat. If you broil a hamburger, it should be cooked thoroughly to the very center of the meat because it contains bacteria all the way into the center. However, solid cuts of beef and lamb should be sterile on the inside. Only the outside needs to be thoroughly cooked to make them safe to eat. Therefore, instructions are given here for cooking steaks and chops to your preference, whether that is well-done or medium-rare.

    Tender cuts of beef steak (T-bone, rib, New York, etc.) or lamb chops
    Dash of salt
    Dash of pepper (optional)

Trim any excess fat from the meat. Score it with a knife at 2-inch intervals around the outside edge to keep it from curling up as it cooks. Place it on a broiler pan. Set the pan in the stove about 3 to 4 inches from the heating unit. Turn the broiler on to 500°F or to the broil setting. Broil the steak(s) or chop(s) until the top of the meat is well-browned. Then turn the meat and broil the other side. For a thin chop or steak to be well done or a 1-inch thick steak to be medium-well, broil the meat for 10 minutes on each side. Season the meat with salt and/or pepper right before serving it.

Broiled Hamburgers

**Gluten-Free IF
buns and toppings are GF**

If you wish to make hamburgers using game meat, you may want to braise rather than broil them so they can be cooked thoroughly without being tough. See the recipe for braised game burgers on page 77 of The Ultimate Food Allergy Cookbook and Survival Guide *which is described on the last pages of this book.*

    1 pound lean ground beef or additive-free* ground turkey
    ½ teaspoon salt
    Dash of pepper (optional)
    4 hamburger buns, wheat-free or gluten-free to fit your diet
    Optional toppings - sliced cheese, tomatoes, lettuce, pickles, catsup,
        mustard, etc.

Mix the beef or turkey, salt, and pepper with your hands. Lightly shape the mixture into four patties. Place the patties on a broiler pan and broil at 500°F about 3 to 4 inches from the heat. Broil the burgers for 10 minutes, then turn them and broil the other side for 10 minutes. Cut one of the burgers to make sure the inside is no longer pink before serving. If it is still pink, cook them a few minutes longer. These burgers will be well done and should not give you an *E. coli* infection. If you shorten the broiling time, you do so at your own risk. Serve the burgers on split buns with the toppings of your choice. Makes four servings.

*Note:** Ground turkey from the grocery store often contains natural flavorings which can be derived from wheat or corn. Ask your health food store to stock additive-free Shelton's ground free range turkey. (See "Special Diet Resources," page 200).

Broiled Fish

Gluten-Free

Fish fillet(s) or steak(s), any kind
Dash of salt.

Put the fish on a broiler pan. Turn the broiler on to 500°F or to the broil setting and broil the fish about 3 to 4 inches from the heating unit. Broil the first side of skinless filets or steaks for five minutes. Turn the fish with a spatula and broil the other side for five minutes. If the fish is thicker than one inch, increase the broiling time to 10 minutes per inch of thickness of the fish. Filets with skin may be broiled skin side down for the whole cooking time. At the end of the broiling time, pierce the fish with a fork to see if it is opaque throughout and flakes easily. If it is opaque throughout and flakes easily, it is done. If not, broil it for an additional few minutes and test it with a fork again. Remove it from the broiler pan and serve it immediately.

Stove Top Poached Fish

Gluten-Free

Orange roughy is a good choice for poaching in either of the next two recipes.

Fish fillet(s) or steak(s), any kind
Water
Dash of salt

Add water to a covered skillet to a depth of ½ to 1 inch, depending on the thickness of the fish. Salt the water lightly and bring it to a boil over high heat. Add the fish, put the cover back on the skillet and let the water return to a boil. Turn the heat down to medium or low and simmer the fish until it is opaque throughout and flakes easily when pierced with a fork. This will take about 10 minutes per inch of thickness of the fish. Serve immediately.

Oven Poached Fish

Gluten-Free

Fish fillet(s) or steak(s), any kind
Water
Dash of salt

Place the fish in a single layer in a glass baking dish. Add water to a depth of ½ inch and sprinkle with salt. Cover the dish with its lid or foil. Bake at 350°F for 15 to 25 minutes (the longer time is for thicker fish), or until the fish flakes easily. Serve immediately.

Quick and Easy Chili

Gluten-Free

1 pound lean ground beef, ground buffalo, or ground red game meat
½ small onion, chopped, or 2 tablespoons chopped dry onion (optional)
1 27-ounce can plus 1 16-ounce can kidney beans
2 16-ounce cans GF tomato sauce
¼ teaspoon salt
½ to 2 teaspoons chili powder, or to taste

Crumble the ground beef into a large saucepan. Cook it over medium-high heat, stirring often, until broken up and no pink color remains. Add the fresh onion, if you are using it, to the pan and cook it with the meat for a few more minutes. Drain off and discard the fat. Drain the liquid from the beans. Add the beans, tomato sauce, dry onions, salt, and chili powder to the pan and heat to boiling. Reduce the heat and simmer it for 5 to 30 minutes. Makes 6 servings. Leftovers freeze well.

Pasta

Gluten-Free IF
GF pasta is used

Pasta is a most versatile main or side dish. If you are gluten-intolerant or allergic to wheat, there are many delicious varieties of wheat-free pasta on the market. (See the "Special Diet Resources" pasta listings on pages 197 to 199). How you cook your pasta can either bring out the best in it or turn it to mush, so follow these basic instructions for cooking it

> 10 ounces to 1 pound of pasta - DeBoles™ rice pasta, quinoa pasta, Purity Foods™ spelt pasta, or other wheat-free or gluten-free pasta
> 3 to 6 quarts of water
> ½ to 1 teaspoon salt

Put the water and salt in a large pot. (The purpose of the salt is to increase the boiling temperature of the water slightly). Bring the water to a rolling boil over high heat. Add the pasta and stir to keep it from sticking together. If you are cooking spaghetti and it is too long for the pan, don't break it. Just put one end into the pan, let it soften a little, and then stir it all in. Return the water to a boil and then reduce the heat slightly to keep the pasta from boiling over while maintaining a good boil. Begin timing the cooking of the pasta from the time the water returns to a boil. Set a large colander in your kitchen sink so you will be ready to drain the pasta when the right time comes.

The best estimate of how long to cook the pasta will be what the package says for cooking time. This varies with the size and shape of the pasta, the type of flour it is made from, and the altitude at which you are cooking. At the minimum cooking time given on the package, take a piece of pasta from the pan and taste it. It should be *al dente* when you bite into it, or offer some resistance to the tooth, without being hard. If it is not done, continue to boil it, retesting it at one to two minutes intervals, until it is done. Then immediately pour it though the colander to drain. Do not run cold water on it. After draining the pasta, put it back into the pan or a serving bowl and toss it with a little oil or pasta sauce to keep it from sticking together. Serve immediately with grated cheese and pasta sauce if desired. Makes 4 to 6 servings.

Dinner's in the Oven

Conventional ovens usually are not considered time-saving appliances, but they can be if you count *your* time rather than just how much time it takes food to cook. Although the food will cook slowly (and have time for the flavors to blend deliciously), the amount of time you spend working on the meal can be brief. The recipes in this chapter include some for your whole meal cooked in one baking pan or casserole and some that are for entrées or side dishes which cook in separate pans but at the same time as parts of an oven meal.

Oven meals usually consist of a main dish, a starchy side dish such as a grain or starchy vegetable, a non-starchy vegetable, and possibly a dessert all baked together in the oven at the same time. When I first tried them, I was amazed at how delicious and easy-to-make oven grains and oven vegetables were – much tastier than their stove-top counterparts. All of these dishes, including the desserts, are more flexible than some oven-baked foods such as pies and cakes. They can cook at a range of temperatures and for a range of times. Whatever the main dish needs, they will take also. However, you may need to add a little more water to them if they will cook for a longer-than-usual time or at a higher temperature. See pages 154 to 155 for dessert recipes that work well with an oven meal.

With your whole dinner in the oven, you can get some real work done or visit with guests in the hour or two before dinner. Serve the side dishes (and maybe even the main dish) directly from the casserole or baking dish they cooked in and you will save time on washing dishes.

One Dish Meals

Fish in Papillote

Gluten-Free

This is an incredibly delicious, no-dirty-dishes meal and is special enough for guests. Don't let the length of the recipe text deter you from trying it! To make it most healthfully, cook the fish and vegetables in a parchment paper pouch. Don't be put off by the detailed directions for making the pouch - it's quick and easy to do and results in great flavor. If you must, you can substitute aluminum foil.

⅓ to ½ pound fish fillets per serving, preferably a mild tasting fish such as orange roughy, tilapia, etc.

Vegetable of your choice, such as 8 to 10 spears of asparagus, 1 to 2
   carrots, or a small piece of broccoli per serving
1 teaspoon oil or butter per serving (optional)
1 teaspoon lemon juice per serving (optional)
Dash of salt
Dash of pepper (optional)
Dash of paprika (optional)

For each serving, cut a piece of parchment paper about twice as long and four times as wide as the fillet of fish. Fold it in half (so it is now twice as long and twice as wide as the fish) and cut it so it will be the shape of a plump heart when opened. Rub the center of the paper with a little of the butter or oil, if you are using it. If you prefer not to use butter or oil, the fish will still taste fine, but it might stick to the paper a little.

Peel the carrots, if you are using them. Cut each carrot into about six thin strips lengthwise. If you are using the broccoli, cut it into thin lengthwise strips. Break off the woody stem ends of the asparagus. Soak and swish them in water to remove any dirt from the tips.

Lay the fish on the parchment paper about ½ inch from the fold. Sprinkle the fish with the optional paprika. Lay the vegetable strips on top of the fish. Drizzle the fish and vegetables with the oil and lemon juice and sprinkle them with the salt and pepper. Preheat your oven to 400°F.

Fold the top half of the parchment paper over the fish and vegetables along the crease that you made to cut the heart shape. Starting at the top center of the half-heart, hold the two cut edges of paper together, fold ½ inch of the edge toward the center of the heart and crease it. Fold this small section of the edge toward the center of the heart and crease it again. Then move a little farther along the edge of the half-heart and fold another small section of the edge of the paper toward the center of the heart twice in the same manner. Each double-folded section should overlap the previous section a little. Keep moving around the heart and folding small sections so that each section anchors the previous section until you reach the point at the bottom of the heart. Twist the paper at the point to lock the whole edge in place.

Put the parchment pouches on a baking sheet. Bake them for about 30 minutes if you are using thin fillets of fish. If you are using thick fillets, open one pouch and make sure the fish is opaque and flakes easily with a fork before serving it; if it is not done, cook the pouches a few minutes longer and then check again. Serve each person's fish and vegetables in the pouch.

Oven Stew

Gluten-Free

2 pounds beef stew meat or beef or buffalo round or chuck steak cut into
    1 to 2 inch cubes
1 onion cut into eighths (optional)
4 carrots, peeled or scrubbed and cut into quarters
4 celery stalks cut into quarters
1 green bell pepper, seeded and cut into one-inch squares
¼ cup quick-cooking (minute) tapioca
1 to 2 cups fresh or 1 8-ounce (drained weight) can of mushrooms,
    drained (optional)
1 teaspoon salt
¼ teaspoon pepper
1 28-ounce can of peeled tomatoes with the liquid
1 cup GF dry red wine or water

Thoroughly stir together all of the ingredients in a large casserole dish with a tight fitting lid such as a Dutch oven, or if you don't have a dish that is large enough, divide the ingredients into two 2½ to 3-quart casserole dishes with lids. Bake at 300°F, covered, for 4 hours. Resist the impulse to open the oven and uncover the stew to check it until near the end of the cooking time. Do check it at about 3 hours after you put it into the oven and add a little more water if needed. Makes 8 to 10 servings. Leftovers freeze well. If your Dutch oven is large enough, you can double the recipe or make a 1½ size batch to have more leftovers to freeze.

Lemon Chicken

Gluten-Free

This is easy yet delicious enough to make for guests.

About 2 pounds of chicken pieces (breasts, thighs or legs) or a 2-pound
    chicken, cut up (skinless saves a little time)
3 to 4 potatoes, or about 1 to 1½ pounds of potatoes
2 tablespoons lemon juice
1½ tablespoons vegetable oil, divided
¼ teaspoon salt
Dash of pepper (optional)
Dash of paprika (optional)
Dash of lemon pepper (optional)

Lightly oil a 13-inch by 9-inch baking dish. Scrub the potatoes and cut them in half lengthwise; then cut each half into three lengthwise wedges. Lay the potato wedges skin side down on one half of the dish. Brush the potatoes with ½ table-spoon of oil and sprinkle them with the paprika, about half of the salt, and pepper if desired. Remove the skin from the chicken and lay the chicken pieces on the other end of the baking dish. In a small bowl, mix together the remaining 1 table-spoon of the oil and the lemon juice. Brush the chicken pieces with the lemon-oil mixture. Sprinkle the chicken with the remaining salt, paprika, and pepper or lemon pepper. Bake the dish at 400°F for 1½ hours, brushing the chicken with the remaining lemon-oil mixture after one hour of baking. Makes 4 servings.

Main Dishes

These main dishes are great as part of an oven meal. Pair them with an oven grain and/or oven vegetable and oven dessert. The oven side dish recipes begin on page 80. The dessert recipes are on pages 154 to 155.

Roast Beef, Lamb, or Pork

Gluten-Free

Roasting should be used as a cooking method only with tender cuts of meat. The less tender cuts may be stewed or cooked in a crock pot for good results. See "Crock Pot Roast Dinner" on page 87.

> Roast of beef, lamb, or pork
> Dash of salt
> Dash of pepper

Place the roast fat side up on a rack in a roasting pan. Season the meat with salt and/or pepper. Turn the oven on to 350°F and put the roast into the center of the oven. Estimate the cooking time at 20 to 30 minutes per pound for beef, depend-ing on how well done you like it, at 30 to 35 minutes per pound for lamb, or at 40 minutes per pound for pork. (In my opinion, pork should always be cooked well-done to kill any eggs of the parasite *Trichinella* which may be present). The actual roasting time depends on the shape of the roast and the fat content of the meat. Therefore, you will need to test your roast with a meat thermometer to see when it is cooked to your preference. Insert the thermometer into the center of the thickest part of the roast, but don't let it touch bone. The final thermometer read-ings should be:

Beef - rare: 140°F
Beef - medium: 160°F
Beef - well done: 170°F
Lamb: 160 to 180°F
Pork: 170 to 180°F

Remove the roast from the oven when it has reached the right internal temperature. Allow it to stand for about 10 to 15 minutes for easier carving.

Pepper Steak

Gluten-Free

1 pound beef or game round steak, cut into serving-size pieces
1 to 2 bell peppers
Dash of salt
Dash of pepper
Water

Remove the stems and seeds from the peppers and slice them into strips. Place the steak pieces into a glass baking dish. Add water almost to the top of the meat. Sprinkle the meat with salt and pepper and top it with the bell pepper strips. Cover the dish with its lid or with foil and bake it at 350°F for 2 hours. As the baking time nears completion, check the steak as it is cooking and add more water if necessary to keep it from drying out completely. The water should have almost completely evaporated by serving time. If it seems to be evaporating too slowly, remove the lid during the last 15 minutes of baking and turn up the temperature if necessary so that the water evaporates and the meat browns. Makes about 4 servings.

Oven Fried Chicken

**Gluten-Free IF
GF flour is used**

3 pounds of skinless chicken breasts or parts of any kind
½ to ¾ cup flour, any kind – rice (GF), cassava meal (GF), barley, spelt, etc.
¼ teaspoon salt
⅛ teaspoon pepper

Skin the chicken and cut it into serving-sized pieces. Combine the flour, salt, and pepper in a plastic bag. Put the chicken pieces into the flour one or two at a time and shake the bag to coat the chicken thoroughly. Place the chicken pieces in a baking dish in a single layer. Turn your oven on to 375°F. Bake the chicken, uncovered, for one hour. Remove the pan from the oven and tilt it to allow the fat to run to one corner of the pan. Use a spoon or baster to pick up the fat and dribble it over the poultry. (If you wish, you can baste the chicken with oil instead of pan drippings). Return the chicken to the oven and bake it for another hour, for a total cooking time of 2 hours. Remove it from the oven when it is browned and crisp. Makes 6 to 8 servings.

Ground Beef Enchilada Casserole

Gluten-Free

1 pound extra lean ground beef
½ of a 1-pound bag of frozen chopped peppers and onions OR
  ¾ cup chopped green bell pepper (about ½ of a large pepper) plus
  ¾ cup chopped red bell pepper (about ½ of a large pepper) plus
  ½ cup chopped onion (optional)
½ to 1 teaspoon chipotle powder or chili powder, to taste (Use the
  smaller amount of chipotle powder with hot salsa).
1 6-ounce can GF tomato paste
3 to 3¼ cups GF bottled salsa, divided
2 to 3 cups shredded cheddar cheese
8 to 12 6-inch corn tortillas

Cook the meat, onion, and peppers in a skillet over medium heat, stirring and breaking the meat up, until the meat is brown throughout and the vegetables are soft. Drain any fat. Add the chipotle powder, 1 to 1¼ cups of the salsa, and the tomato paste to the meat mixture and simmer about 5 to 10 minutes longer. Reserve ½ cup of the cheese.

Preheat your oven to 350°F. Spread ½ cup of the salsa on the bottom of a 3-quart casserole dish. Top with a layer of slightly overlapping tortillas. (Depending on the size and shape of the dish, you may have to cut the tortillas to fit the dish). Top the tortillas with half of the meat mixture, half of the non-reserved cheese, and one third of the remaining salsa. Repeat with another layer of tortillas, meat, cheese, and salsa. Top with a final layer of tortillas and the remaining salsa. Cover the dish with foil or its lid and bake for 30 to 45 minutes or until it is heated through. Remove the foil or lid, sprinkle with the reserved cheese, and bake for another 5 minutes or until the cheese is melted. Makes 4 to 6 servings.

Oven Side Dishes

Oven Grains

Gluten-Free IF
made with a GF grain

These grains are easy to prepare yet so delicious that they make an oven meal special.

Brown rice (GF):
> 1 cup brown rice
> 2½ cups water
> ½ teaspoon salt, or to taste
> 1 tablespoon oil
>> Cooking time: 1 to 1½ hours

White rice (GF):
> 1 cup white rice
> 2½ cups water
> ½ teaspoon salt, or to taste
> 1 tablespoon oil
>> Cooking time: 1 to 1½ hours

Wild rice (GF):
> 1 cup wild rice
> 4 cups water
> ½ teaspoon salt, or to taste
> 1 tablespoon oil
>> Cooking time: 1½ to 2 hours

Quinoa (GF):
> 1 cup quinoa
> 2½ cups water
> ½ teaspoon salt, or to taste
> 1 tablespoon oil
>> Cooking time: 1 hour

Millet (GF):
> 1 cup millet
> 3½ cups water
> ½ teaspoon salt, or to taste
> 1 tablespoon oil
>> Cooking time: 30 to 45 minutes

Sorghum/Milo (GF):

1 cup sorghum (milo)
3½ cups water
1 tablespoon oil
½ teaspoon salt, or to taste
> Cooking time: 2½ to 3 hours

Buckwheat (GF):

1 cup white or roasted buckwheat groats
3½ cups water
½ teaspoon salt, or to taste
1 tablespoon oil
> Cooking time: 1 to 1½ hours

Teff (GF):

1 cup teff
3 cups water
½ teaspoon salt, or to taste
1 tablespoon oil
> Cooking time: 1 to 1½ hours

Oat Groats*:

1 cup oat groats
2¾ cups water
½ teaspoon salt
1 tablespoon oil
> Cooking time: 2 hours

Rye:

1 cup rye
3¾ cups water
½ teaspoon salt
1 tablespoon oil
> Cooking time: 2 hours

Spelt:

1 cup spelt
3½ cups water
½ teaspoon salt
1 tablespoon oil
> Cooking time: 2 to 2½ hours

Pearled or hulless barley:

> 1 cup pearled or hulless barley
>
> 3½ cups water
>
> ½ teaspoon salt, or to taste
>
> 1 tablespoon oil
>
> > Cooking time: 2 to 2½ hours for pearled barley, 1½ hours to 2 hours for hulless barley

Kamut:

> 1 cup kamut
>
> 3½ cups water
>
> 1 tablespoon oil
>
> ½ teaspoon salt
>
> > Cooking time: 1¾ to 2 hours

Choose one set of ingredients from the list above. If you are cooking quinoa, be sure to rinse it in a strainer under running water until the water is no longer sudsy to remove its natural soapy coating. Combine all of the ingredients in a 2 to 3-quart glass casserole dish with a lid. Cover the dish and bake at about 350°F until the grain is tender and all the water is absorbed. The baking time is flexible so these grains can usually be baked the same amount of time as the entrée of an oven meal. Approximate baking times for each type of grain are given at the end of each ingredient list above. If you will be baking the grain for much longer than these times or at a higher temperature, you may need to add a little more water. Check it near the end of the cooking time the first time you make it and make a note of how much extra water you added if it was needed. Makes about 2 cups of cooked grain or 4 half-cup servings.

*Note: Ask your doctor if oats are allowed on your gluten-free diet.

Oven Carrots

Gluten-Free

This dish will make you a cooked carrot lover, especially if made with whole organic carrots.

> 2 to 2½ pounds whole carrots or pre-peeled mini carrots
>
> ⅓ cup water
>
> ½ teaspoon salt
>
> 2 to 3 tablespoons oil

If you are using pre-peeled mini carrots, bake them at 350°F in a covered casserole dish for an hour. Drain off the water at this point in the recipe.

If you are using whole carrots, peel or scrub them and cut them lengthwise into quarters or into eighths if they are very large. Lay the carrot sticks parallel to each other in a 2 to 3 quart glass casserole dish with a lid.

To the partially cooked mini carrots or the raw whole carrot sticks, add the salt and water and drizzle the oil over the top of the carrots. Cover the dish with its lid and bake carrot sticks at 350°F for about 1 to 1½ hours or mini-carrots for an additional hour, or until they are browning and becoming caramelized. Makes 6 to 12 servings.

Oven Cabbage

Gluten-Free

1 head of cabbage weighing about 1½ to 1¾ pounds
½ teaspoon salt
¼ teaspoon pepper (optional)
⅓ cup water
3 tablespoons oil

Coarsely chop the cabbage and put it into a 3-quart glass casserole dish with a lid. Add the salt, pepper, and water. Drizzle the oil over the top of the cabbage. Cover the dish with its lid and bake at 350°F for 1 to 2 hours, stirring mid-way if you are at home. Makes 6 to 9 servings.

Easy Baked Vegetables

Gluten-Free

These are the easiest starchy foods to have with your oven entrée.

White potatoes, white or orange sweet potatoes, or winter squash

Scrub and pierce the potatoes. Cut the squash in half and remove the seeds. Place the squash cut side down on a baking dish or a baking sheet with an edge. You may place white potatoes directly on the oven rack. Orange sweet potatoes sometimes ooze sticky liquid so you may wish to use a baking dish for them. Bake with the rest of your oven meal for 1 to 2½ hours at 350°F to 450°F or until they are tender when squeezed and your main dish is done. (Use a longer cooking time with the lower temperatures). An average serving size is one-half pound of squash or one potato per person.

Oven Peas or Beans

Gluten-Free

Because you start with frozen vegetables, this is very quick and easy to prepare.

1 10-ounce package frozen peas, cut green beans, or lima beans
⅓ cup water
⅛ teaspoon salt
1 tablespoon oil

Combine all of the ingredients in a 1 to 1½ quart glass casserole dish. Cover the dish with its lid, and bake at 350°F for 1 to 1½ hours for the beans or 20 minutes to 1 hour for the peas. Makes 2 to 4 servings.

Oven Onions

Gluten-Free

1½ pounds of small onions
Water
Salt
1 tablespoon of oil (optional)

Peel the onions and put them into a 3-quart casserole dish. Add water to ¼ inch depth and cover the dish with its lid or aluminum foil. Bake at 350°F for 40 to 50 minutes or up to 1½ hours until they are tender or done to your preference, or cook them until the rest of your oven meal is done. (For longer baking times, add water to ½ inch depth). Drain off the water. Season with salt and drizzle with a little oil before serving if desired. Makes 6 to 10 servings.

Special Oven Squash

Gluten-Free

The easiest way to prepare winter squash in the oven is to cut it in half, remove the seeds, and bake it cut side down. (See page 83). However, if you have a little extra time and would like a change from plain squash, this is very tasty.

2½ pounds butternut squash
¼ teaspoon salt
2 tablespoons oil

Peel the squash. Cut it in half lengthwise and remove the seeds. Slice it into ¼-inch slices. Put the slices into an 11 inch by 7 inch baking dish, sprinkle them with the salt, and drizzle them with the oil. Stir to coat all of the slices. Bake at 350°F for 1½ to 2 hours, turning the slices after the first hour. Makes 6 to 9 servings.

Crispy Oven Sweet Potatoes or White Potatoes

Gluten-Free

It is quickest to just scrub, pierce and bake potatoes, but if you want to make a special dish and have time for slicing, these potatoes are delicious.

> 1½ pounds white potatoes or 2 pounds sweet potatoes
> 2 tablespoons oil
> ½ teaspoon salt
> Pepper to taste (optional; it is great with the white potatoes)

Peel or scrub the potatoes and slice them into ¼-inch slices. (Sweet potatoes are best peeled). Put the slices into an 11 inch by 7 inch baking dish, sprinkle them with the salt and optional pepper, and drizzle them with the oil. Stir to coat all of the slices. Bake at 350°F for 1½ to 2 hours, turning the slices after the first hour. Makes 4 to 8 servings.

Dinner's in the Crock Pot

If you are on a special diet and short on money or time, a crock pot can be a lifesaver. With a crock pot, you can start your dinner before you leave in the morning and have a delicious meal waiting for you when you get home. A crock pot will save you money because less expensive cuts of meat are flavorful and tender when cooked all day and because dried beans are easily prepared in a crock pot.

The recipes in this chapter are the right size for a three-quart crock pot. If your crock pot is not that size, you can still use these recipes. If you are cooking for one or two people, cut the recipes in half for smaller size crock pots. However, I would advise investing about $20 to $25 in a larger crock pot to make the best use of your time. If you cook more of these crock pot dishes than you will eat immediately, you can freeze the leftovers for future meals. When you take the leftovers out of the freezer on a busy day, you will be glad that you did it. The very best way to use a crock pot to simplify your life is to purchase a five to six-quart crock pot, double the recipes in this chapter, and freeze enough leftovers for several meals.

The bean soups in this chapter take little time to make, but you will have to plan ahead and start the recipe the night before you want to eat them. Put the beans to soak overnight. If you will be in a rush the next morning, also prepare the vegetables and other ingredients. In the morning, rinse the beans, add the other ingredients to the pot, turn it on, and you will have a delicious, wonderful smelling dinner ready to eat when you come home.

Meat Dishes

Corned Beef Dinner

Gluten-Free

This is an easy meal that offers a change from the ordinary for family and guests.

    1 2 to 3-pound corned beef brisket
    2 to 3 potatoes, scrubbed or peeled and cut into large chunks
    3 to 4 carrots, scrubbed or peeled and cut into 2-inch pieces
    Water
    1 head of cabbage (optional)
    ½ teaspoon salt
    Dash of pepper (optional)

Scrub or peel and cut up the carrots and potatoes and put them into the bottom of a three quart crock pot. Place the corned beef on top of the vegetables. If the corned beef spices come in a separate package, sprinkle them over the meat. Add water to the crock pot until it is almost to the top of the meat. Cook on low heat for 10 to 12 hours or on high heat for 5 to 8 hours. About a half hour before dinner time, cut the cabbage into wedges. Fill a large saucepan about ⅔ full of water and bring it to a boil. Add the cabbage wedges, salt, and pepper and boil until the cabbage is cooked to your preference. Drain the cabbage. Remove the brisket from the crock pot and slice it against the grain. For guests, arrange the meat and vegetables on a platter to serve. Makes 4 to 6 servings.

Crock Pot Roast Dinner

Gluten-Free

This recipe makes inexpensive, less-tender cuts of beef taste like gourmet fare. It's so easy and delicious that it makes a great meal to cook for company. With most of the meal in your crock pot, you will have time to really enjoy your guests.

1 2 to 2½-pound chuck roast, rump roast, or pot roast of beef, buffalo, or other red game meat
2 large or 3 small potatoes, scrubbed or peeled and cut into chunks (optional)
3 carrots, scrubbed or peeled and cut into 2-inch pieces
1 onion, peeled and sliced or cut into eighths (optional)
½ cup water, GF beef broth, or GF red wine
1 tomato, chopped, 1 tablespoon GF tomato paste, or 2 to 3 tablespoons GF catsup (optional)
Dash of salt
Dash of pepper (optional)

Scrub or peel and cut up the vegetables and put them into the bottom of a three quart crock pot. Set the roast on top of the vegetables. Stir together the water, broth, or wine with the tomato, tomato paste or catsup. Pour the liquid over the roast. Sprinkle the roast with the salt and pepper. Cook on low for 10 to 12 hours or on high for 5 to 8 hours. This recipe is very tasty when made with a sweet red wine such as Marsala. The alcohol evaporates during cooking leaving just its flavor, but if you are allergic to yeast, do not use the wine. If you prefer more juice with your roast, increase the amount of water, broth or wine to 1 cup and double the amount of tomato, tomato paste or catsup. Makes 4 to 6 servings.

Sauerbraten

Gluten-Free IF
gravy not made with spelt

This is an impressive dish to serve to guests although it involves a little more work than the previous crock pot recipes. Serve it with mashed or baked potatoes.

1 2 to 3-pound rump roast
1¼ cups water, divided
1 cup wine vinegar
1 tablespoon salt
2 tablespoons Fruit Sweet™ or honey OR ¼ cup apple juice concentrate,
    thawed
1 medium onion, sliced (optional)
1 unpeeled lemon, sliced
10 whole cloves
4 bay leaves
10 whole peppercorns
3 tablespoons tapioca starch (GF), arrowroot (GF), or corn starch (GF)
    OR ¼ cup white spelt flour (optional – for gravy)

A day or two before you plan to serve this recipe, put the meat into a deep glass bowl or casserole dish. Stir together 1 cup of the water, the vinegar, salt, and sweetener. Pour them over the meat. Add the onion, lemon, cloves, bay leaves, and peppercorns to the liquid around the meat. Refrigerate for 24 to 36 hours, turning the meat once or twice during the marinating time. The morning of the day you plan to serve this, remove the meat from the liquid and put it in a 3-quart crock pot. Add 1 cup of the marinating liquid to the crock pot. Discard the rest of the marinating liquid. Cover the pot and cook it on low for 8 to 10 hours or on high for 5 to 8 hours. Remove the meat from the pot and put it on a serving platter. If you wish to have gravy with this meal, stir the starch or flour thoroughly into the remaining ¼ cup of water until any lumps are gone. (Lumps will not be a problem with the starch; if you use the flour, a hand blender will get rid of the lumps). Pour the liquid from the crock pot into a saucepan. Add the starch or flour-water mixture to the pan and cook it on the stove over medium heat for a few minutes until it comes to a boil and thickens. Serve the gravy with the meat. Makes 4 to 6 servings.

Crock Pot Stew

Gluten-Free

2 pounds stew meat or round or chuck steak or of any kind - beef,
    buffalo, lamb, or red game meat
5 carrots (about 1 pound)
3 stalks of celery
1 onion (optional)
1½ pounds of potatoes (about 3 or 4, optional)
½ cup quick-cooking granulated or minute tapioca
2 bay leaves (optional)
2 teaspoons salt
¼ teaspoon pepper (optional)
2¼ cups water OR 1 28-ounce can peeled tomatoes

If you are using steak rather than stew meat, trim the fat and gristle from the meat and cut it into one or two inch cubes. Scrub or peel the carrots and potatoes. Cut the carrots into one inch pieces and cut the potatoes into two inch chunks. Slice the celery into one inch slices. Put the meat, vegetables, tapioca, seasonings, and water or tomatoes into a 3-quart crock pot. Stir the stew thoroughly to evenly distribute the tapioca. Cook it on low for 8 to 12 hours or on high for 5 to 6 hours. If you like your stew juicy, check the stew about 1 hour before the end of the cooking time and add a little boiling water if needed. Makes 6 to 8 servings. If made without the potatoes, this stew freezes well. The potatoes may become mushy if they are frozen.

Poultry Dishes

Turkey Breast Dinner

Gluten-Free

This meal is so easy that you can throw it in the crock pot in five minutes before leaving for work without any preparation the night before.

1 1-pound bag pre-peeled mini carrots
1 10-ounce package frozen cut green beans
1 to 1½ pounds turkey breast (boneless skinless for the least work) or
    turkey tenders
1 tablespoon water
¼ to ½ teaspoon salt, or to taste
Dash of pepper (optional)
Dash of paprika (optional – for color)

Pour the carrots into the bottom of a 3-quart crock pot. Pour the green beans on top. Lay the turkey breast on top of the beans. If you purchased turkey breast with the bones and skin, you may either remove the skin before putting it in the crock pot or, for maximum moistness of the meat, remove it after cooking. If your turkey will not fit into the pot easily with the bones, break or cut them with kitchen shears so you can bend and fit the breast in the crock pot. Sprinkle the 1 tablespoon water over the turkey. Then sprinkle the turkey and vegetables with the salt and pepper. Sprinkle only the turkey breast with paprika. Cook on the low setting for 8 to 10 hours. Makes 4 servings. Leftovers freeze well.

Chicken Fricassee

**Gluten-Free IF
spelt flour not used**

This meal is low in fat and freezes well. Although it takes a little time to remove the chicken from the bones, it's worth it for the great low-fat nutrition.

> 1 2 to 3-pound chicken, skinned and cut into pieces, or skinless chicken
>   breasts or other meaty chicken pieces
> 1 teaspoon salt
> ½ teaspoon paprika (for color – optional)
> 1 small onion, sliced (optional)
> 3 stalks of celery, sliced
> 3 to 5 carrots, peeled and sliced (about 1 pound)
> 1 bay leaf
> 2 cups water or GF chicken broth
> ¼ cup additional water
> ¼ cup tapioca starch (GF), arrowroot (GF), cornstarch (GF), or white spelt
>   flour

Put the onion, celery, carrots, and bay leaf in a 3-quart crock pot. Place the chicken pieces on top of the vegetables and sprinkle them with the salt and paprika. Pour the 2 cups of water or broth into the pot. Cover and cook on low for 8 to 12 hours or on high for 4 to 5 hours. Remove the chicken pieces. Turn the crock pot to high. Thoroughly combine the ¼ cup water with the flour or starch and stir the mixture into the vegetables and liquid in the pot. Remove the chicken meat from the bones and skin. Discard the bones and skin. When the liquid in the pot has thickened, return the chicken meat to the pot and cook for a few minutes more to reheat the chicken. Add more boiling water to the pot if you like your fricassee more juicy. Serve over hot noodles or cooked rice or other grain. (See recipes on pages 73, 80, and 126). Makes 6 to 8 servings. Leftovers freeze well.

Bean Soups

Multi-Bean Soup

Gluten-Free

This soup takes 20 minutes of your time to make – 5 minutes the evening before you want to eat it, 10 minutes the next morning, and 5 minutes near serving time. If you're pressed for time in the morning, the time required can be 10-5-5 minutes instead. This soup is delicious, nutritious and economical as well as quick.

> 1 pound mixed dry beans (Check that the mix does not contain barley).
> Water
> ½ pound peeled mini-carrots or 3 to 5 whole carrots
> 3 stalks of celery
> 1½ to 2 teaspoons salt, to taste
> ¼ teaspoon pepper (optional)
> 1 15-ounce can diced tomatoes (optional)

The evening before you want to have this soup for dinner, put the beans in a strainer and run water over them thoroughly to remove any dirt. Put them in a 3-quart crock pot and fill the pot nearly full with water. Soak them overnight. If you are pressed for time in the morning, prepare the carrots and celery at this time as described below. Store the prepared vegetables in a container or plastic bag in the refrigerator overnight.

In the morning, drain the water from the crock pot by holding the lid very slightly ajar and pouring the water off through the crack between the lid and the pot. Refill the pot with water and drain it two times more.* Add 5 cups of water to the pot and turn it on to high. If you are using peeled mini-carrots, you may add them to the pot whole or cut them in half. (Using mini-carrots straight from the bag instead of whole carrots will save you about 5 minutes of time). If you are using whole carrots, scrub or peel them and slice them into ½ inch slices. Wash the celery, lay the stalks together on a cutting board, and slice all three stalks into ½ inch pieces at the same time. Add the carrots and celery to the crock pot. Cook the soup on high for 5 to 6 hours or, if you are leaving for the day, turn it down and cook it on low for 8 to 10 hours.

When the beans are tender (if cooked on high for 5 to 6 hours), or slightly before serving time (if cooked on low), add the salt, pepper, and tomatoes. If you are not using the tomatoes and the soup seems too thick, add up to 1 cup of boiling water. If you are adding the tomatoes shortly before dinner time, warm them in the microwave before adding them to the pot.

This recipe makes about 2½ quarts of soup, or 5 to 8 servings. If you want to make a larger batch to freeze, use a 5-quart crock pot, double the amounts of all of the ingredients, and cook the soup on high for 8 to 10 hours. A double batch makes about 5 quarts of soup, or 10 to 16 servings.

*Note: Rinsing the beans after soaking them removes indigestible carbohydrates that can cause intestinal gas.

Black Bean Soup

Gluten-Free

This spicy soup gives dinner some pizzazz.

> 1 pound dry black beans
> Water
> 2 bell peppers, preferably one red and one green, seeded and diced
> 1 small onion, diced (optional)
> 1 teaspoon ground cumin (optional)
> 2 teaspoons salt
> ½ teaspoon pepper or a 2 inch chili pepper, seeded and crumbled
> 2 teaspoons dry oregano
> 1 15-ounce can diced tomatoes or 1 pound tomatoes, chopped

The night before you plan to serve this soup for dinner, rinse the beans by running water over them in a strainer to remove any dirt. Put them in a 3-quart crock pot and cover them with cold water. Soak them overnight. If you are pressed for time in the morning, chop the peppers and onions at this time and refrigerate them in a plastic bag.

In the morning, drain the water from the beans, add fresh water to the pot, and drain the water again. Rinse the beans this way three times.* Drain off all the water after the last rinse. Add 4 cups of water to the crock pot plus the peppers, onion, cumin, salt, pepper, and oregano. Cover the crock pot with its lid and cook the soup on high for 6 hours or on low for 8 to 10 hours. Add the chopped tomatoes an hour before the end of the cooking time, or microwave them to warm them and add them a few minutes before serving time. If the soup is thicker than you prefer, near the end of the cooking time add a little boiling water to the pot. Makes about 2½ quarts of soup, or 6 to 8 servings. Leftover soup freezes well.

*Note: Rinsing the beans after soaking them removes indigestible carbohydrates that can cause intestinal gas.

Navy Bean Soup

Gluten-Free

1 pound dry navy beans
Water
2 carrots
3 stalks celery
2 teaspoons salt
¼ to ½ teaspoon pepper (tastiest with ½ teaspoon, but if you're not into
        hot food, sample it after adding ¼ teaspoon to decide how much to
        add)
1 tablespoon dry parsley
1 teaspoon dry sweet basil
1 potato, peeled and grated (optional)

The night before you plan to serve this soup for dinner, rinse the beans by running water over them in a strainer to remove any dirt. Put them in a 3-quart crock pot and cover them with cold water. Soak them overnight. If you are pressed for time in the morning, prepare the carrots and celery at this time as described below and refrigerate them in a plastic bag.

In the morning, drain the water from the beans, add fresh water to the pot, and drain the water again. Rinse the beans this way three times.* Drain off all the water after the last rinse. Scrub or peel the carrots aand cut them into ¼ inch slices. Lay the celery stalks together and cut the bunch of celery all at once into ¼ inch slices. Add 6 cups of water to the crock pot plus the carrots, celery, salt, pepper, parsley, and sweet basil. Cover the crock pot with its lid and cook the soup on high for 6 hours or on low for 8 to 10 hours. Add the optional potatoes two hours before the end of the cooking time. Check the soup near the end of the cooking time and add a little boiling water to the pot if the soup is thicker than you prefer. Makes about 2½ quarts of soup, or 6 to 8 servings. If made without the potatoes, leftover soup freezes well.

*****Note:** Rinsing the beans after soaking them removes indigestible carbohydrates that can cause intestinal gas.

Split Pea Soup

Gluten-Free

1 pound split peas
Water
3 to 4 carrots
3 stalks celery
2 teaspoons salt
¼ teaspoon pepper
1 bay leaf
1 to 2 cups cubed cooked ham (optional)

The night before you plan to serve this soup for dinner, rinse the peas by running water over them in a strainer to remove any dirt. Put them in a 3-quart crock pot and cover them with cold water. Soak them overnight. If you are pressed for time in the morning, prepare the carrots and celery at this time as described below and refrigerate them in a plastic bag.

In the morning, drain the water from the peas, add fresh water to the pot, and drain the water again. Rinse the beans this way three times.* Drain off all the water after the last rinse. Scrub or peel the carrots aand cut them into ¼ inch slices. Lay the celery stalks together and cut the bunch of celery all at once into ¼ inch slices. Add 5 cups of water to the crock pot plus the carrots, celery, salt, pepper, ham, and bay leaf. Cover the crock pot with its lid and cook the soup on high for 6 hours or on low for 8 to 10 hours. Check the soup near the end of the cooking time and add a little boiling water to the pot if the soup is thicker than you prefer. Remove the bay leaf before serving. Makes about 2½ quarts of soup, or 6 to 8 servings. Leftover soup freezes well.

*Note: Rinsing the peas after soaking them removes indigestible carbohydrates that can cause intestinal gas.

Lentil Soup

Gluten-Free

Because lentils are probably the least allergenic legume, it you omit the optional tomatoes and pepper, this soup is the bean soup most likely to be tolerated by those with extensive food allergies.

> 1 pound dry lentils
> Water
> 3 to 5 carrots
> 3 stalks celery
> 2 teaspoons salt
> ¼ teaspoon pepper (optional)
> 1 15-ounce can diced tomatoes (optional)

The night before you plan to serve this soup for dinner, rinse the lentils by running water over them in a strainer to remove any dirt. Put them in a 3-quart crock pot and cover them with cold water. Soak them overnight. If you are pressed for time in the morning, prepare the carrots and celery at this time as described below and refrigerate them in a plastic bag.

In the morning, drain the water from the lentils, add fresh water to the pot, and drain the water again. Rinse the beans this way three times.* Drain off all the water after the last rinse. Scrub or peel the carrots aand cut them into ¼ inch slices. Lay the celery stalks together and cut the bunch of celery all at once into ¼ inch slices. Add 5 cups of water to the crock pot plus the carrots, celery, salt, and pepper. Cover the crock pot with its lid and cook the soup on high for 6 hours or on low for 8 to 10 hours. Add the optional tomatoes an hour before the end of the cooking time. Check the soup near the end of the cooking time and add a little boiling water to the pot if the soup is thicker than you prefer. Makes about 2½ quarts of soup, or 6 to 8 servings. Leftover soup freezes well.

*Note: Rinsing the lentils after soaking them removes indigestible carbohydrates that can cause intestinal gas.

Dinner's in the Freezer

This book contains many recipes that freeze well and can be made in large batches. Harried but wise cooks will use such recipes to stock their freezers with meals to have ready to eat on future busy days. The recipes below are those that just ask to be made in large batches and frozen. (How else are you going to use up all that zucchini?) Near the end of the chapter you will find some recipes that require more effort, so I like to make them in large batches and freeze them. They include pasta sauce and lasagne recipes which allow my family to stay in touch with our Italian roots in spite of a busy lifestyle. A list of the best freezer recipes in the book can be found on page 103.

Zucchini Stew

Gluten-Free

My grandma made this with ground beef but if you are eating a low-fat diet or are allergic to beef, try ground turkey, buffalo or other game meat. This is one of the rare recipes in which zucchini freezes well. If you have an overflow of zucchini from your garden, double, triple or even quadruple the recipe and freeze most of what you make.

> 2 tablespoons chopped onion or 1½ teaspoons dry chopped onion (optional)
> 1 pound lean ground beef, turkey, buffalo, or other game meat
> 1 15 or 16-ounce can of peeled tomatoes with the juice
> 1 8-ounce can of GF tomato sauce OR ⅜ cup (about half of a 6-ounce can) of GF tomato paste plus ¼ cup water
> ½ teaspoon salt
> ¼ teaspoon pepper (optional)
> 2 to 2½ pounds of zucchini sliced about ⅜ inch thick

If you wish to use fresh onion, combine it with the meat in a large saucepan. Cook the meat mixture over medium heat, stirring occasionally, until the meat is brown. Pour off the fat to discard. Add the tomatoes, tomato sauce or tomato paste plus water, dry onion, salt, and pepper. Return the mixture to a boil over medium to high heat. Reduce the heat and simmer it for about 15 minutes. (If you are using game meat, simmer it longer until the meat is tender. Add more water if it begins to dry out). Add the zucchini, return the stew to a boil, reduce the heat, and simmer for an additional 10 to 15 minutes or until the zucchini is just tender. (Large zucchinis take longer to cook than small ones). Add an additional ¼ cup of water if the stew begins to dry out or is thicker than you prefer. Makes 4 to 6 servings.

Economy Chili

Gluten-Free

This recipe is very economical as well as great to have in your freezer for future meals. My original version is not very hot. My son Joel, who is a time-pressed graduate student, makes his chili more exciting by substituting salsa for the tomato sauce and adding jalapeno peppers and crumbled dry chili pequin peppers for heat and flavor. (See "Sources," page 213 if you cannot find chili pequin peppers locally). When I discussed using this recipe as a time-saver with Joel, he said it doesn't take him much total time to make but he does plan ahead to soak the beans the night before he makes it and to spend a few minutes on various steps of the recipe at the needed times the next day.

> 1 pound dry kidney beans
> Water
> 1½ to 2 pounds of lean ground beef, buffalo, or other red game meat
> 1 12-ounce can GF tomato paste
> 1 16-ounce can GF tomato sauce (For Joel's hot chili, substitute 2 cups of salsa).
> 1 small onion, chopped, or 3 tablespoons dry chopped onions (optional)
> 1 teaspoon salt
> 1 to 3 teaspoons of chili powder, to taste, or 5 to 6 crumbled 1-inch long dried chile pequin peppers (Use the chile pequin for Joel's hot chili).
> 1 to 2 4-ounce cans sliced jalapeno peppers, drained, or 2 to 5 fresh jalapeno peppers, chopped (optional – Use with seeds for hot chili).

The evening before you plan to serve the chili, rinse the beans by running water over them in a strainer to remove any dirt. Put them in a 3-quart crock pot and cover them with cold water. Allow the beans to soak overnight.

Preparation of the meat can be done the evening before if you will not be home an hour or two before dinner, or it can be done the afternoon of the day you serve this recipe. In a separate pan on the stove, brown the ground meat. Add the optional fresh onion and fresh jalapeno peppers and cook for a few minutes more. Drain and discard the fat. If you are doing this the evening before, refrigerate the meat mixture. If you want to eat quickly when you get home the next day, warm it in the microwave oven before adding it to the crock pot. If you have more time to let the flavors meld, you can add it to the crock pot cold an hour or two before serving time.

In the morning, drain the water from the beans, add fresh water to the pot, and drain the water again. Rinse the beans this way three times. (This soaking and rinsing process removes difficult-to-digest carbohydrates which can cause intestinal gas). Add enough water to the beans in the pot to cover them. Cook on high for 4 to 6 hours or on low for 8 to 10 hours.

When the beans are tender, drain the water until it is at about half of the level of the beans in the pot. Stir the tomato paste into the pot thoroughly. Add the cooked meat, dry onions, tomato sauce or salsa, canned jalapeno peppers, and seasonings. If you like your chili juicer, add some boiling water and drain less of the bean cooking liquid the next time you make this recipe. If you are adding these ingredients shortly before dinner, cook on high for 10 to 20 minutes. If you have more time, the flavor will be best if you can cook the chili for another 1 to 2 hours on high. Makes 6 to 8 to servings.

If you wish to make a larger batch of this chili in a 5-quart crock pot, multiply the amounts of the ingredients by 1½.

Traditional Pasta Sauce with Meatballs

Gluten-Free

Before you question whether this recipe is made "with ease," some information about authentic Italian pasta sauces is in order. Southern Italians make their pasta sauces quickly and flavor them with garlic and spices. The flavor in Northern Italian pasta sauces is developed by long, slow cooking. This recipe is a take-off on my grand-mother's Northern-type recipe and originally involved cooking the meatballs in a frying pan with frequent tending and turning and then stirring the sauce every ten minutes for half of the day. The rest of the day could be spent cleaning up sauce spatters from anywhere within ten feet of your stove. Therefore, this recipe really is much easier than my grandmother's way of making sauce. Although you have to be home for the initial part of the cooking time, the recipe does not require the constant attention of the original recipe and there are no spatters to clean up.

Sauce ingredients:

> 1 28-ounce can GF tomato puree
> 3 6-ounce cans GF tomato paste (or 1 12-ounce can plus 1-6 ounce can)
> ½ to 1 teaspoon salt
> ⅛ to ¼ teaspoon pepper (optional)
> ⅝ cup water*

Meatball ingredients:

    2 pounds of lean ground beef, buffalo, or other red meat
    1 teaspoon dry parsley (optional)
    ½ teaspoon salt
    ¼ teaspoon pepper (optional)
    1 clove of garlic, peeled and chopped (optional)

Open the cans of tomato puree and paste and scrape their contents into a 3-quart crock pot using a rubber spatula. Add the ⅝ cup water*. Thoroughly stir together the sauce ingredients to eliminate the tomato paste lumps. Turn the pot to the high setting and let the sauce begin heating while you prepare the meatballs. If you like a southern Italian flavor to your pasta, you may also add ½ teaspoon dry oregano and ½ teaspoon dry sweet basil to the sauce at this point.

Preheat your oven to 400°F while making the meatballs. In a 13 by 9 inch cake pan or glass baking pan or on a rimmed baking sheet (like a jelly roll pan), combine the meat, salt, pepper and parsley for the meatballs. Use your hands to mix the ingredients together thoroughly. Form the meat into 8 meatballs, pressing the meatballs together firmly with your hands. Arrange the meatballs in the pan so they have at least one inch of space between them. Sprinkle the pieces of the optional clove of garlic in the baking pan.

Put the pan in the oven and bake for 15 minutes. Remove the pan and turn the meatballs with a spatula. Put the pan into the oven for another 15 minutes. Remove the meatballs from the pan and put them in the crock pot. Push them down into the sauce so they are submerged. Traditionally, in my family, the garlic was discarded at this point. (If cooked with the meat and discarded, it just scents the sauce). However, if you want a more garlicky Southern Italian flavor, add the garlic to the sauce. Drain the fat from the baking pan into a can to discard.

Turn the temperature control on the crock pot to low and allow the sauce to cook for several more hours or for 8 to 10 hours total cooking time. Or, if you will be at home and want to shorten the cooking time and/or have thicker sauce, you may cook it on high for 4 to 6 hours after adding the meatballs. If you are cooking the sauce on high, every 1 to 1½ hours stir the sauce gently being careful not to break the meatballs. Use a rubber spatula for stirring because it will not cut the meatballs and you can scrape the sides of the pot well with it. If you will be at home for just one or two hours after adding the meatballs to the sauce, you can cook it on high for that time. When you must leave, or after the sauce has thickened, stir the sauce and turn the temperature down to low until dinner time. You do not need to stir it when it is on low. Serve the sauce with cooked pasta. (See the recipe for cooking pasta on page 73).

This recipe makes about 5 cups of sauce and 8 meatballs, enough sauce for 2 pounds of pasta or for two meals, or 6 to 8 servings. Leftovers freeze well. If you are serving this to company, it simplifies your entertaining to make the sauce a few days or weeks ahead and freeze it. My dad always said the sauce tasted better the second time he ate it – after it had been in the freezer for a while. This recipe can be doubled and cooked in a 5-quart crock pot, which is a great way to stock your freezer for future easy meals.

*Note: Traditionally, my family's sauce recipes measured the water in "cans of water" rather than measuring cup amounts. To save getting out a measuring cup to measure ⅝ cup of water, you may add one small can of water from the 6-ounce tomato paste can to this recipe. One less utensil to deal with saves a little time.

"Meatballs the Old Way" variation:

My family is very particular that their Italian food be just like it has always been. They find meatballs cooked in the oven as in this recipe dry. Therefore, to make sauce for them, I use 2½ pounds of regular ground beef rather than using lean ground beef and cook the meatballs the traditional way rather than baking them. To cook them the traditional way, form the meat mixture into balls with your hands and put them in a frying pan on medium heat. Turn them as they cook until all sides are well browned. If you wish to use the garlic but do not want to add it to the sauce for more potent garlic flavor, add the garlic to the frying pan whole. It is easier to remove this way. I also cook the sauce on high and remove the meatballs after the sauce has been boiling 1 to 1½ hours because all-day cooking makes the meatballs seem slightly different to my family (although still basically all right).

Lasagne

Gluten-Free

Any lasagne recipe takes some time to make, but this version made with a crock pot and no-boil pasta is quicker and easier than most. This is an ideal dinner for a special celebration because it can be made a day or a month ahead, and while it is in the oven, you can enjoy your party.

Sauce ingredients:

> 2 pounds lean ground beef, buffalo, or other meat
> 2 12-ounce cans GF tomato paste
> 1 28-ounce can GF tomato puree
> 1½ cups water
> 1 teaspoon salt
> ⅛ teaspoon pepper (optional)

Additional ingredients:

> 1½ to 2½ 10-ounce boxes of no-boil rice lasagne noodles such as DeBole's™
> 3 15 to 16-ounce containers of ricotta cheese
> ½ cup grated Romano or Parmesan cheese
> 1 32-ounce package of mozzarella cheese
> 1½ tablespoons chopped dried parsley (optional)

Start making the sauce early in the morning on a day when you have adequate time to cook if you want to serve, refrigerate, or freeze the lasagne that evening. Or, if you want to spread the work out a little, make the sauce at least one day before you plan to serve, refrigerate, or freeze the lasagne.

Combine the tomato paste, tomato puree, water, salt and pepper in a 3-quart crock pot and turn it on to the high setting. Cook the meat in a frying pan over medium heat, breaking it up and stirring it often, until it is well browned. Pour off the fat into a can to discard. Add to the meat the crock pot and stir thoroughly. If you are having the lasagne the next day or later, you may turn the temperature control on the crock pot to low and allow the sauce to cook unattended for 8 to 10 hours total cooking time. Or, if you will be at home and want to shorten the cooking time and/or have thicker sauce, you may cook it on high for the four to six hours, stirring it every 1 to 1½ hours. Cooking the sauce on high will allow you to assemble the lasagne the same day that you make the sauce.

The sauce may be refrigerated overnight or frozen. Makes about 2½ quarts of sauce. If you wish to make lasagne often, make a double batch of sauce in a 5-quart crock pot and freeze what you do not use. When you want to make more lasagne, the sauce will be ready to go and you can make just the number of pans you need that day.

Lasagne assembly instructions:

In a bowl, combine the ricotta cheese, Romano or Parmesan cheese, and parsley. Mash them together with a potato masher. Slice the mozzarella cheese thinly.

Spread about 1½ to 2 cups of the sauce (total amount for all pans) over the bottoms of a 13 inch by 9 inch cake pan or a similar-sized deep casserole dish plus a 2½ to 3-quart casserole dish. If you do not need a large pan for guests, use three 2½ to 3-quart casserole dishes. Lay dry lasagne pasta in a single layer over the sauce. (The amount of pasta you need will vary with the type of baking dishes you are using as well as with the thickness of the noodles). Spread the pasta with about 3 to 3½ cups of the sauce. Layer about half of the mozzarella cheese over the sauce. Spread about half of the ricotta mixture over the mozzarella. Add another layer of pasta to the dish, followed by another 3 to 3½ cups of sauce, the rest of the mozzarella, and the rest of the ricotta mixture. Add a third layer of pasta to the dish and top it with about 2 cups of sauce. Serve any remaining sauce on the side with the lasagne. If you wish to, you may refrigerate or freeze the lasagne at this point. Cover the dish with plastic wrap to refrigerate or freeze it.

When you are ready to bake the lasagne, thaw it completely in the refrigerator if it has been frozen. Cover it with aluminum foil or with the lid of the casserole dish. Put the lasagne into your oven and turn it on to 350°F. Bake it for about 1½ hours or until it is hot throughout and bubbly at the edges. If you refrigerated or froze the lasagne before baking it, allow about an extra ½ hour or more of baking time. If it was frozen and is not completely thawed before baking it, you will have to add even more baking time. Makes 12 to 15 servings or enough lasagne to have guests once and save a meal for four people in the freezer.

RECIPES WHICH ARE IDEAL FOR FREEZING:

Almost all of the main and side dish recipes as well as the baking recipes in this book can be frozen, but the recipes listed below are especially good for making in large batches and using to stock your freezer so you always have pre-made meals on hand for dinner.

Quick and Easy Vegetable Soup, page 113
Multi Bean Soup, page 91
Black Bean Soup, page 92
Navy Bean Soup, page 93
Split Pea Soup, page 94
Lentil Soup, page 95
Oven Stew, page 76
Crock Pot Stew, page 89 (Omit the potatoes).
Chicken Fricassee, page 90
Quick and Easy Chili, page 72
Economy Chili, page 97
Zucchini Stew, page 96
Traditional Pasta Sauce with Meatballs, page 98
Lasagne, page 101

Microwave Marvels

Microwave ovens make it much easier to save time in the kitchen. However, they are not as standardized as conventional ovens. They vary in size, power, and whether they contain a turntable. Therefore, the cooking times for the recipes in this chapter are also more variable and are given as a time range. The first time you use a recipe, cook it for the shortest time given. If it is not done at that time, check it in another minute or two until it is cooked to your satisfaction. Then write down the cooking time in this book so you will know how long to cook it the next time.

Microwave ovens are wonderful for heating up leftovers or meals you have taken from your freezer. (See pages 37 to 38 about freezer meals and freezing conventionally cooked entrées). However, I advise against using them to cook meat-containing main dishes unless you are cooking ground meat that can be stirred because it is possible to have cold spots that never cook thoroughly. This could lead to food safety problems. See "In-a-Hurry Chili," page 105, for the only meat-containing microwave recipe in this book.

Vegetables are ideal foods for the microwave. If you are pressed for time or pressed for space on your stove top, consider cooking vegetables in the microwave. Most bags of frozen vegetables give microwave cooking instructions on the bag. Follow these instructions, because frozen vegetables vary in how long they should be cooked depending on how much blanching or pre-cooking they underwent before being frozen. To cook fresh vegetables in the microwave, see the recipes on pages 106 to 112.

My mother-in-law was the first family member to purchase a microwave oven when they were the latest thing in time-saving cooking equipment. She was excited at the idea of being able to cook much more quickly, but then discovered that my father-in-law did not like the taste of many foods prepared in the microwave. However, she managed to save some time anyway by microwaving potatoes until they were partially cooked and then finishing the cooking process in the oven, and my father-in-law ate them without complaining. She told me, "Do it this way and they'll never know the difference."

As I was pondering how to cook more quickly when developing recipes for this book, I wondered if her part microwave-part conventional cooking method would work for other vegetables. It does! The carrot recipes on pages 106 to 107 taste much better than stove top-cooked carrots but are ready much more quickly than "Oven Carrots," page 82. These microwave-plus-conventional recipes can be cooked in the oven or broiler at the same time as your entrée.

In-a-Hurry Chili

Gluten-Free

If you are in a real hurry and need dinner for only one or two people, see the note on how to make a small batch extra quickly at the end of this recipe.

1 pound lean ground beef
3 8-ounce cans GF tomato sauce
3 15-ounce cans kidney beans
¼ teaspoon salt
½ to 1 teaspoon chili powder, or to taste

Crumble the ground beef into a hard plastic colander set in a large casserole dish. Microwave on high for 5 to 8 minutes, stirring and breaking up the meat every 2 minutes, until the meat no longer has any pink spots. Drain the grease from the casserole and discard. Add the cooked meat and tomato sauce to the casserole, cover it with the lid or plastic wrap, and microwave on high for 5 minutes. Drain the liquid in the can from the beans and add them to the casserole dish. Add the seasonings and microwave on high for another 5 to 7 minutes, stirring every 2 to 3 minutes. Makes 3 to 8 servings.

Note: To make a large serving for one or two medium-sized servings more quickly, use ⅓ pound ground beef, 1 can of tomato sauce, 1 can of beans, and a dash of salt, and chili powder to taste. Microwave the meat for 3 to 5 minutes, the meat and tomato sauce for 5 minutes, and all of the ingredients together for another 5 minutes.

Speedy Mashed Potatoes

Gluten-Free

These are especially delicious when prepared with Yukon Gold potatoes.

1 to 1¼ pounds Yukon Gold or white potatoes*
1 tablespoon water
1 to 2 tablespoons oil or butter
1 tablespoon milk or water
Salt and pepper to taste

Thoroughly scrub the potatoes. Put them in a glass casserole dish with a lid. Add 1 tablespoon of water to the dish, put the lid on, and microwave on full power for 10 to 15 minutes. Add the butter, additional 1 tablespoon of water or milk, salt, and pepper. Mash with a potato masher. Makes 2 to 3 servings.

Note: This recipe is best made with thin-skinned potatoes. Russet potatoes can be used if they're what you have on hand, but the skin will be more obvious to fussy eaters.

Microwave Plus Vegetable Recipes

Nuke-n-Bake Potatoes

Gluten-Free

This is the way to get "real" baked potato texture in much less time.

> 4 large baking potatoes

Preheat your oven to 450°F while you are cleaning and microwaving the potatoes. Scrub the potatoes and pierce them with a knife in several places. Arrange the potatoes in a circle on the turntable of your microwave and cook them on full power for 4 minutes. Turn them over and cook them for another 4 minutes. The potatoes should be starting to feel soft when squeezed by this time. If they are not, microwave them for a few more minutes. Transfer them to the conventional oven and bake them for another 12 to 15 minutes. You will have "real" baked potatoes in only about 25 minutes or less.

Nuke-n-Bake Carrots or Glazed Carrots

Gluten-Free

Carrots prepared by long baking in the oven are so delicious that once you have eaten them, you will not want steamed or boiled carrots ever again. However, there will be days when you do not have enough time to prepare "Oven Carrots" (recipe on page 82). This recipe and the next provide two microwave-plus-conventional recipes that approximate the taste of oven carrots in much less time.

> 1 pound peeled mini-carrots
> ¼ cup water
> ¼ teaspoon plus a dash of salt
> 2 to 3 teaspoons oil
> 1 tablespoon agave, Fruit Sweet™ or honey (optional)

Put the carrots in a flat glass baking dish or 1-quart casserole dish with ¼ cup of water and ¼ teaspoon of salt. Cover and microwave on high for 8 minutes. Preheat your oven to 500°F (or whatever temperature your entrée requires) while they are microwaving. If possible, stir them after the first 4 minutes of microwaving. (The microwave time may vary with the power of your microwave and how well done you like your vegetables). Drain the carrots. Drizzle them with the oil and sprinkle them with salt to taste. For glazed carrots, also drizzle them with the agave, Fruit Sweet™ or honey. Stir and arrange the carrots so they are mostly in one layer. Bake uncovered at 350°F to 500°F for ½ to 1½ hours, using higher temperatures with shorter baking times. If you wish you may stir them mid-way through the baking time if you will be around to do so; if you are baking them hot and fast, stirring is recommended. The longer you bake them, the more they will caramelize. Makes 3 to 4 servings.

Nuke-n-Broil Carrots

Gluten-Free

This is a great way to cook carrots if you have your broiler heated to cook steaks or broil fish.

1 pound peeled mini-carrots
¼ cup water
¼ teaspoon plus a dash of salt
2 to 3 teaspoons oil

Put the carrots in a glass baking dish with ¼ cup of water and ¼ teaspoon of salt. Cover and microwave on high for 8 minutes. If possible stir them after the first 4 minutes of microwaving. (The microwave time may vary with the power of your microwave and how well done you like your vegetables). Drain the carrots and put them into an 8 or 9 inch square metal cake pan, drizzle them with the oil and sprinkle them with salt to taste. Stir and arrange the carrots so they are mostly in one layer. Broil at 500°F for 10 minutes. They will have begun to brown and can be eaten at this point if desired. However, if you have time to cook them longer, stir and re-arrange them and then broil them another 5 to 10 minutes or until they are well-browned. Makes 3 to 4 servings.

Nuke-n-Bake Winter Squash

Gluten-Free

The hardest part of cooking many winter squashes is cutting them in half before you bake them. This recipe makes that easy.

1 large winter squash weighing about 3 pounds

Pierce the squash with a knife in at least two places making sure that you go all the way into the center cavity. This keeps it from exploding in the microwave. Cook it in the microwave on full power for 8 minutes. Cut the squash in half and remove the strings and seeds. Place the halves cut side down in a glass baking dish and microwave for another 4 minutes. Preheat your oven to 450°F while the squash is microwaving. Transfer the squash to the oven and cook it for another 15 minutes. Drier types of winter squash, such as kobacha, will be more mealy when cooked this way than if just microwaved. Makes about 6 servings.

Microwaved Fresh Vegetables

Here are instructions for cooking the more common fresh vegetables in the microwave. These recipes do not included some vegetables, such as corn cut from the cob, beans, and peas, because if you are short on time, you will want to use frozen corn, beans, and peas rather than stringing, cutting, and shucking fresh vegetables. To cook frozen vegetables, follow the instructions on the bag. To cook less commonly eaten fresh vegetables, see the "Vegetable Primer" chapter in *Easy Cooking for Special Diets* as described on the last pages of this book.

Asparagus

Gluten-Free

Hold both ends of each asparagus stalk and bend. Discard the root end. Swish the stalks in a sink of cold water, allowing a little soaking time to loosen any dirt that might be hiding in the tips. If there is any dirt or grit in the bottom of the sink, change the water and swish again until the grit is all removed. Take the asparagus from the water. If desired, cut the stalks into one-inch pieces.

For whole spears, arrange them in a glass baking dish with the tip ends lined up down the center of the dish. Add ¼ cup of water. Cover with a lid or plastic wrap and microwave on high for 6 to 9 minutes for 1½ pounds (purchased weight rather than prepared weight) of asparagus. Let stand one minute; drain and serve. For one inch pieces, put the asparagus in a glass casserole. Add ¼ cup of water. Cover and microwave for 6 to 9 minutes for 1½ pounds of asparagus, stirring every 3 minutes. Serve with butter or oil and salt if desired. Makes about 4 servings.

Broccoli

Gluten-Free

Trim off any leaves and cut the stems to about 4 inches in length. Wash the broccoli and cut it into spears by cutting downward between the stalks making sure that the stalks are not thicker than ½ inch. If desired, cut off the florets and cut the stalks into one inch pieces.

To cook spears, arrange the broccoli in a square or rectangular baking dish with the florets lined up down the center of the dish. Add 1 cup of water for 1½ pounds of broccoli. Cover the dish with plastic wrap and microwave on high for 10 to 14 minutes or until the broccoli is tender or almost tender. Let it stand for 5 minutes; then drain the water. Makes about 6 servings.

To cook broccoli pieces, put the pieces in a casserole dish and add 1 cup of water for 1½ pounds of broccoli. Cover the dish with plastic wrap and microwave on high for 10 to 14 minutes or until the broccoli is tender or almost tender. Let it stand for 5 minutes; then drain the water. Makes about 6 servings.

For one to two servings, prepare the broccoli as above but use about 5 to 6 ounces of broccoli, ½ cup of water, microwave on high for 5 to 7 minutes, let it stand for 5 minutes; then drain the water.

Serve with a little butter or oil and salt and/or pepper if desired.

Cabbage

Gluten-Free

Cut a small (¾ to 1 pound) head of cabbage into wedges or core it and shred it or cut it into squares. Put it in a 2 quart casserole dish with ¼ cup of water and ½ teaspoon of salt. Cover it and microwave it on high for 6 minutes. Stir the shredded or cut-up cabbage or rearrange the cabbage wedges so that what was in the center of the casserole is at the edge. Cover and microwave the cabbage on high for another 4 to 8 minutes. Let it stand for 3 to 5 minutes. Drain and serve with oil and salt if desired.

Cauliflower

Gluten-Free

Wash the cauliflower and remove the outer leaves. Cut off any dark spots from the florets. Cut the florets from the center core. Put the florets from one medium (about 1 pound) head of cauliflower in a 1½ quart casserole dish with ¼ cup of water and ¼ teaspoon of salt. Cover and microwave on high for 5 minutes. Stir, cover, and microwave until tender, another 4 to 8 minutes. Drain and serve with a little butter or oil and salt if desired.

Corn on the Cob

Gluten-Free

Corn on the cob is best very fresh. As soon as it is picked, the natural sugars begin to convert to starch and it looses sweetness, so try to eat your corn soon!

Fresh ears of corn
Water
Plastic wrap or parchment paper

Remove the husks from the corn and break or cut off the stem (if present). Remove any tassel strings that cling to the corn by wiping the ear with a damp piece of paper towel from the narrow tip of the ear to the end where the husk was attached. Rinse each ear. If you are not going to cook the corn right away, dry each ear and refrigerate them in a plastic bag.

For each ear of corn, cut a 12 inch square piece of plastic wrap or a 13 inch square piece parchment paper. If the corn is dry, rinse it again or put about 1 teaspoon of water on the wrap or paper. If you are using plastic wrap, lay the corn diagonally on the wrap. Fold one corner of the wrap over the corn, fold down the corners near the ends of the ear, and roll the corn up in the remaining plastic wrap. If you are using parchment paper, lay the corn in the middle of the paper parallel to one of the sides. Fold one half of the paper over the top of the corn so the cut edges come together. Fold and roll the cut edges together until you reach the corn. Then twist the ends of the paper at the ends of the ear of corn.

Put the corn on the turntable of the microwave and microwave on high for 3 minutes for one ear, 5 minutes for two ears, or 8 minutes for four ears. If you cook four ears at once, half-way through the cooking time, rearrange them on the turntable so that the ears that were in the center are on the outside and the ears that were on the outside are in the center. The cooking time can vary with the power of your microwave, altitude, etc.

Let the corn stand for a minute or so before eating it. If the cob seems mushy, decrease your cooking time next time. If the corn is not done, microwave it a minute or two longer and increase your cooking time next time.

Spinach and Other Greens

Gluten-Free

If you do not have time for washing spinach but prefer fresh to frozen for cooking, buy the pre-washed bagged spinach that is sold with the salad greens. This recipe can also be used for other greens such as collards, kale, chard, etc.

Remove the stem ends from the spinach or greens. Put the leaves in a sink filled with cool water and swish them around. Lift them out into the other side of the sink, fill the sink with water, and swish them again. Repeat this several times until there is no more dirt left in the water when you lift the greens out. If you are using pre-washed spinach, it (obviously) does not need to be washed. Just put it in the sink with water to get it wet before proceeding with this recipe.

Place 1 pound of greens in a 3 quart casserole dish with the water from washing them still clinging to the leaves. Cover and microwave on high for 3 minutes. Stir, cover, and microwave until tender, another 3 to 5 minutes. Let stand 3 minutes. Drain and serve with a little butter or oil and salt if desired.

Squash – Summer

Gluten-Free

Use this recipe to cook zucchini or crookneck squash.

Wash the squash and cut about ¼ inch off of each end. Cut it into ½ inch thick slices. Put the squash slices in a 1½ quart casserole dish with ¼ cup of water and ¼ teaspoon of salt. Cover and microwave on high for 4 minutes for 1½ pounds of squash. Stir, cover, and microwave until tender, another 3 to 7 minutes. Let stand for one minute, drain and serve with a little butter or oil and salt if desired.

Squash – Winter

Gluten-Free

There are so many delicious varieties of winter squash! Try them all until you find your favorites.

Pierce squash with a knife in at least two places, being sure to go all the way into the center cavity. Place the whole squash in the microwave oven. For 2 pounds of squash (about one medium squash), microwave on high for 6 minutes. Cut the squash in half and remove the seeds and strings. Arrange the halves cut-side down in a baking dish. Cover and microwave on high for 6 to 9 minutes more or until the squash is tender when pierced with a fork. Allow it to stand for 3 minutes before serving. Serve with a little butter or oil and salt or honey if desired.

Sweet Potatoes

Gluten-Free

Sweet potatoes are often called yams although they are really in a different food family than true yams. They come in all colors from pale yellow to orange to red. The yellow or "white" sweet potatoes are less sweet and more mealy.

Scrub the potatoes under running water. Pierce with a fork in several places to keep them from exploding in the microwave oven. Put a piece of paper towel on the turntable of your microwave oven. Arrange the sweet potatoes in a circle on the paper towel, spacing them at least two inches from each other. Microwave on high until tender when pierced with a fork. This will be about 5 minutes for one potato or about 12 minutes for 4 potatoes, with varying times between for two or three potatoes. Allow the potatoes to stand for 5 minutes before serving with butter or oil and salt.

White Potatoes

Gluten-Free

Baked potatoes can be made very quickly in the microwave. If you want the texture of oven-baked potatoes, see "Nuke-n-Bake Potatoes" on page 106.

Scrub the potatoes under running water. Pierce with a fork in several places to keep them from exploding in the oven or microwave oven. Arrange the potatoes in a circle on the turntable of your microwave, spacing them at least two inches from each other. Microwave on high until tender when pierced with a fork. This will be about 5 minutes for one potato or about 12 to 15 minutes for 4 potatoes, with varying times between for two or three potatoes. Allow the baked potatoes to stand for 5 minutes before serving with butter or oil and salt.

Satisfying Soups

Soup makes a delicious and economical cold-weather meal. But what kind of soup? Quick soup usually means canned food laden with strange ingredients and excess sodium and which may not be especially nutritious. Real soup is delicious homemade soup which nourishes both body and soul. However, it can involve hours of work in the kitchen. The soup recipes in this book fall into a third category. They are homemade and nutritious but can be made easily with minimum time and effort.

The soup recipes in this chapter will be ready quickly. (Those in the crock pot chapter on pages 91 to 95 cook all day in the crock pot, but they require little or no attention from you while they are cooking). A few of the recipes in this chapter call for beef or chicken broth. Get a brand from your health food store that is made from natural foods rather than from ingredients which may be harmful, allergenic, or contain gluten. See pages 202 to 204 for some of these brands.

Pair the soup recipes below and on pages 91 to 95 with a salad, bread, muffins or crackers, and some fresh fruit for dessert and you will have a satisfying meal which supplies great nutrition at low cost.

Quick and Easy Vegetable Soup

Gluten-Free IF made with rice

This large batch of soup makes a great meal plus plenty of delicious leftovers for your freezer.

> 6 cups of GF beef broth (See pages 202 to 204).
> 1 14 to 16-ounce can of diced tomatoes
> ¼ cup quick-cooking barley or white rice
> 1 10-ounce package of frozen mixed vegetables (peas, beans, carrots, and corn)*
> 1 small stalk of celery, sliced
> 1 small onion, chopped, or 3 tablespoons dry chopped onion (optional)
> ¼ head of cabbage, chopped
> 2 to 3 cups of cubed cooked beef, such as leftover roast

Combine the beef broth, tomatoes and rice or barley in a large pot and bring the soup to a boil over high heat. When it comes to a boil, reduce the heat to low and simmer for 5 minutes. Add the frozen vegetables, celery, and onion, raise the heat, and bring the soup back to a boil. Reduce the heat and boil the soup gently for 10 more minutes. Add the cabbage and beef and bring the soup back to a boil. Reduce the heat and boil gently for another 5 minutes. Makes about 8 servings.

*Note: If you are allergic to corn, use a package of peas and carrots instead of the mixed vegetables.

Corn Chowder

Gluten-Free

This soup is quick, easy, and flavorful. To make it even quicker, omit the optional vegetables or use dry chopped onion, and the only thing you will have to chop is the potato.

> 2 tablespoons oil (Use it only with the celery and/or fresh onion).
> ⅓ stalk celery to make about ¼ cup diced celery (optional)
> 1 jalapeno pepper, 2 to 4 tablespoons chopped green chili pepper, or 2 to 4 tablespoons canned jalapeno or chopped green chili pepper, to taste (optional)
> ¼ cup fresh chopped onion, 1 tablespoon dry chopped onion, or an additional ⅓ stalk or ¼ cup diced celery (optional)
> 4 cups of water or GF chicken broth (See pages 202 to 204).
> 1 tablespoon lemon juice (optional)
> 1 teaspoon salt (Omit if you use broth; use only if you use the water).
> ⅛ to ¼ teaspoon pepper, to taste
> 1 large or 2 small potatoes to make 3 cups cubed potatoes
> 1 pound frozen corn

Slice the partial stalk(s) of celery lengthwise into three or four strips. Lay all the strips together and slice them crosswise into about ¼-inch dice. Chop the optional jalapeno or chili pepper and fresh onion. Combine the oil, celery, chili or jalapeno pepper, and fresh onion in a large saucepan. Cook them over medium heat until the vegetables are soft. Scrub or peel the potato(es) and cut them into cubes about ½ inch in size. When the celery, onions, and fresh pepper are cooked, add the rest of the ingredients to the pan with them.

Bring the soup to a boil over medium-high heat. Reduce the heat and simmer the soup for 10 to 15 minutes or until the potatoes are tender. Remove about 3 cups of the soup and puree it with a hand blender, blender, or food processor. Return it to the pot and reheat the soup before serving it. Makes 4 to 6 servings.

This soup does not freeze well. If you cannot eat this large of a batch in a few days, halve the amounts of all of the ingredients.

Streamlined Corn Chowder: Omit the oil, celery, chili or jalapeno pepper, and fresh onion. Scrub the potato(es) to save time. Cut them into cubes about ½ inch in size. Use dry onion if desired and combine it with the last six ingredients in a large saucepan. Proceed with the directions in the second paragraph on the previous page.

Cauliflower and Cottage Cheese Soup
Gluten-Free

The cottage cheese and milk in this soup are great quick sources of protein.

> 1 tablespoon oil (optional – use it only with fresh onion)
> 1 small onion, chopped, or 2 to 3 tablespoons dry chopped onion
>   (optional)
> 3 to 4 cups of chopped fresh cauliflower or 1½ pounds frozen cauliflower
> 2 cups GF chicken broth (See pages 202 to 204).
> 1 cup skim, low fat, or whole milk
> 1 cup low fat cottage cheese
> Dash of salt and pepper, to taste (optional)

If you wish to use the fresh onion, combine it with the oil in a saucepan. Cook it over medium heat until the onion is soft, about 3 minutes. When the onion is cooked, add the cauliflower and broth to the pan and bring it to a boil over medium-high heat. If you are not using fresh onion, just combine the cauliflower and broth in the pan with or without the optional dry onion and bring it to a boil. Reduce the heat and simmer the soup for ten minutes or until the cauliflower is tender. While the cauliflower is cooking, combine the cottage cheese and milk and puree them with a hand blender, blender or food processor until they are smooth. When the cauliflower is cooked, remove about half of the cauliflower and a little of the broth from the pot and puree them with a hand blender, blender or food processor. Return the pureed cauliflower to the pot and add the cottage cheese puree. Reheat the soup gently over low heat, stirring frequently, until it is just under the boiling point. Do not boil. Taste the soup and season with pepper and, if needed, salt to taste. Makes 4 servings.

Potato Soup

Gluten-Free

You can make this soup without the milk if you are allergic to dairy products.

2 medium potatoes, about 1 pound
1 small onion, chopped, or 2 to 3 tablespoons dry chopped onion
    (optional)
1¾ cups water or 1 cup water plus ¾ cup milk (any type of milk you
    tolerate)
¾ teaspoon salt
⅛ teaspoon pepper
Chopped parsley for garnish (optional)

Peel the potatoes. Cut one potato into quarters and the other into ½-inch cubes. Combine the potatoes and onion with the water in a saucepan. Bring them to a boil over medium-high heat; then reduce the heat and simmer them until they are tender, about 20 to 30 minutes. Remove the potato quarters and about ½ cup of the water from the pan and puree them with a hand blender, standard blender or food processor until smooth. Add the potato puree, milk (if you are using it), salt, and pepper to the pan with the potato cubes. Reheat the soup carefully over low heat, stirring frequently, until it is just under the boiling point. If you used the milk, do not let the soup boil. Serve immediately. Makes 2 servings. This recipe may be doubled or tripled to serve more people. It does not freeze well.

Quick Cream of Pea Soup

Gluten-Free

1 16-ounce bag frozen peas
1¼ cups water
1 bay leaf (optional)
¾ teaspoon salt
1 cup milk (any kind you tolerate) or additional water

Put the peas, bay leaf, and water in a saucepan on high heat and bring it to a boil. Turn the heat down to medium and cook for 2 to 4 minutes. Remove the bay leaf from the pan. Puree the peas and water in the pan with a hand blender, or use a standard blender or food processor. Stir in the salt and milk or additional water and reheat the pan carefully on medium heat. If you used the milk, do not allow it to boil. When the soup is steaming, serve it. Makes 4 cups of soup or about 3 servings.

Simple Salads and Dressings

Salads bring two things to mind – superior nutrition and lots of washing and chopping of vegetables. Commercially pre-washed and prepared salad greens or mixes, if not mostly iceberg lettuce, deliver the nutrition minus the washing and chopping. Some people on special diets may find commercially-made salad dressing they tolerate by reading labels carefully in the health food store, but others will not. If you must avoid fermented foods such as vinegar due to yeast allergy, you will probably have to make your own dressing. The dressing recipes in this chapter provide multiple non-vinegar options for tartness, can be made easily, and are delicious on pre-washed packaged salad greens. Because you can double or triple the dressing recipes (except the avocado dressing) you will not have to make dressing often. Just keep some dressing ready in your refrigerator at all times. When you want a salad, toss your homemade dressing with pre-washed salad greens, and dinner will be ready in no time.

Tossed Salad

**Gluten-Free IF
made with GF crackers**

This salad is a powerhouse of nutrition when made with greens or lettuce other than iceberg lettuce. The more darkly colored the greens, the more nutritious. Try pre-washed blends that contain red leaf lettuce, endive, spinach or arugula in this salad.

> 4 cups of leaf lettuce or other greens, any variety or combination, torn into bite-sized pieces
> ¼ to ½ cup sliced carrots, cucumbers, and/or radishes
> 1 medium or large tomato, cut into eight to twelve pieces
> Optional additions to make the salad more substantial:
> > ¼ cup crumbled crackers that are allowed on your diet
> > 2 tablespoons chopped nuts
> > ½ to 1 avocado, peeled and cut into cubes
> > 2 tablespoons crumbled or grated cheese or goat cheese, if tolerated
> > ⅓ cup cooked beans, such as garbanzo beans, drained
> ¼ to ⅓ cup of any salad dressing (commercially made GF dressing or made using the recipes on pages 121 to 123)

Tear the lettuce or greens into bite sized pieces and put them in a large salad bowl. Slice the cucumbers, carrots, or radishes and cut up the tomato; add them to the salad bowl and toss. Add the dressing and toss. Sprinkle the top of the salad with the optional additions such as crackers, nuts, avocado, beans, or cheese. Serve immediately. Makes 2 to 3 servings.

Spinach Salad

Gluten-Free IF made with GF crackers

Pre-washed spinach makes this salad a snap.

> 4 cups of spinach leaves, washed and torn into bite-sized pieces
> 1 cup diced or sliced cooked beets (optional)
> 1 avocado, peeled, seeded, and cut into bite-sized pieces (optional)
> 2 slices of leftover cooked bacon, crumbled (optional, if tolerated)
> ¼ cup of "Oil and Vinegar Dressing," page 121, or similar commercially made GF dressing
> ¼ cup broken crackers that are allowed on your diet (optional)

Put the spinach in a large salad bowl. Slice or cut up the beets or avocado and add the pieces to the salad bowl. Crumble the optional bacon, add it to the salad bowl and toss the salad. Add the dressing and toss. Sprinkle the top of the salad with the crumbled crackers if desired. Serve immediately. Makes 2 to 3 servings.

Coleslaw

Gluten-Free

If you use packaged shredded cabbage, this salad will be ready in a jiffy.

> 1 pound of shredded cabbage or coleslaw mix
> ¼ teaspoon salt (optional)
> ¾ cup GF mayonnaise (commercially prepared or homemade, recipe on page 125) or super smooth sauce, page 124
> 2 tablespoons lemon juice or ¼ teaspoon unbuffered vitamin C powder

Stir together the salt, mayonnaise, and lemon juice or vitamin C in a large bowl. Add the coleslaw mix or shredded cabbage and toss thoroughly until the cabbage is completely coated with the dressing. Makes 6 to 8 servings. Keeps well in the refrigerator.

Make-Ahead Tossed Salad

Gluten-Free IF
made with GF crackers

This is an easy salad that you can make ahead of time when you have a large crowd of guests. For a small party, cut the recipe in half.

½ cup oil, preferably walnut or canola because they are high in essential
   fatty acids
1 clove of garlic, crushed (optional)
½ teaspoon dried oregano, sweet basil or parsley (optional)
½ teaspoon salt
Dash of pepper
⅓ cup wine or apple cider vinegar or lemon juice
½ to 1 cup sliced carrots, cucumbers, and/or radishes
2 to 3 medium tomatoes, each cut into eight pieces
12 cups of leaf lettuce or other greens, any variety or combination, torn
   into bite-sized pieces
Optional additions to make the salad more substantial:
   ¾ cup crumbled crackers
   ⅓ cup chopped nuts
   ⅓ tablespoons crumbled or grated cheese
   ¾ cup cooked beans such as garbanzo beans, drained

If you wish to use the garlic, crush it and put it in the oil in a glass jar. Refrigerate at least overnight. Remove the garlic from the oil and discard the garlic. Combine the oil with the rest of the seasonings and vinegar or lemon juice in a large salad bowl or 4-quart mixing bowl. Stir the dressing thoroughly. Add the carrots, cucumbers, radishes, and tomatoes to the dressing in the bowl. (They will prevent the lettuce from being immersed in the dressing before serving time). Put the lettuce and/or other greens on top of the cut vegetables. Cover the bowl with plastic wrap and refrigerate it until serving time. At serving time, toss the salad. Sprinkle the top of the salad with the crackers, nuts, cheese, and/or beans. Makes 8 to 10 servings. For a small party, cut the recipe in half.

Three Bean Salad

Gluten-Free

The salt-free varieties of canned beans often do not contain sugar or additives. If you can find canned beans you can eat, the preparation of this salad is a breeze.

1¼ cups cooked cut green beans or 1 15-ounce can green beans, drained
1 15-ounce can kidney beans, drained
1 15-ounce can garbanzo beans, drained
2 tablespoons chopped onion or 1 to 2 teaspoons dry onions (optional)
½ cup chopped green pepper (optional)
2 tablespoons apple juice concentrate, thawed
¼ teaspoon salt
⅛ to ¼ teaspoon pepper (optional)
⅓ cup lemon juice, apple cider vinegar or wine vinegar OR 2 teaspoons
    tart-tasting unbuffered vitamin C powder, as tolerated (See the
    comment on bowel tolerance below).
¼ cup oil

Combine the beans, onion, and green pepper in a large bowl. In a separate small bowl, stir together the apple juice, lemon juice or vinegar (if you are using either of them), salt, and pepper until the salt is dissolved. Pour this mixture and the oil over the beans, toss them thoroughly, and refrigerate until serving time. (This salad tastes best if the flavors soak into the beans for an hour to overnight). If you are using the vitamin C powder, stir them into 2 tablespoons of water until they dissolve and add them to the salad just before serving. Vitamin C loses its tang in this salad if added very long before serving time. Also, if a large serving is eaten, some individuals do not have bowel tolerance for this amount of vitamin C. Makes 4 to 6 servings.

Dressings

Oil and Vinegar Salad Dressing

Gluten-Free

Because they are not heated, salad dressings are a great place to add fragile oils which are high in essential fatty acids to your diet. Canola and walnut oils are good sources of omega-3 fatty acids which most of our diets lack in sufficient quantities.

½ cup oil, preferably walnut or canola because they are high in essential
    fatty acids
½ teaspoon dried oregano, sweet basil or parsley (optional)
½ teaspoon salt
Dash of pepper
⅓ cup wine vinegar, apple cider vinegar, or lemon juice OR 1 to
    1½ teaspoons unbuffered vitamin C powder plus 1 tablespoons water

Combine all of the ingredients in a jar and shake. The dressing may be refrigerated at this point. Shake the dressing again to thoroughly mix it right before pouring it on your salad. Makes about ¾ cup of dressing. Refrigerate leftover dressing.

Sweet Vinaigrette

Gluten-Free

½ cup oil, preferably walnut or canola because they are high in essential
    fatty acids
½ teaspoon salt
Dash of pepper (optional)
⅓ cup wine vinegar, apple cider vinegar, or lemon juice OR
    1 to 1½ teaspoons unbuffered vitamin C powder (to taste)
    plus 1 tablespoon water
2 tablespoons thawed fruit juice concentrate (apple, pineapple, orange, or
    white grape) or 1 tablespoon agave, Fruit Sweet™ or honey

If you are using the vitamin C, mix it with the water in a glass jar until it is dissolved. Add the rest of the ingredients to the jar and shake. Shake the dressing thoroughly to mix it right before pouring the dressing on your salad. Makes about 1 cup of dressing. Refrigerate leftover dressing.

Avocado Dressing

Gluten-Free

This dressing is delicious on spinach or sliced cucumbers.

> 1 large ripe avocado (about ½ to ¾ pound in weight)
> 2 tablespoons wine vinegar, apple cider vinegar, or lemon juice OR 1
>   teaspoon unbuffered vitamin C powder (or more to taste)
> ⅛ teaspoon salt
> Dash of pepper
> Water

Peel and seed the avocado. Put the avocado flesh in a 2-cup or larger glass measuring cup and mash it slightly or blend it with a hand blender. You should have about ⅔ cup of avocado flesh. Add the lemon juice, vinegar or vitamin C, salt, and pepper to the cup. Add water to the 1 cup mark. Puree with a hand blender until the dressing is smooth. (You can use a standard blender or food processor instead). Serve immediately. This dressing may darken if it stands for very long. Makes 1 cup of dressing.

Creamy French Dressing

Gluten-Free

If you can use the QuickThick™ or ThickenUp™ (which contain corn), this dressing is especially quick and easy to make.

> ¼ cup water
> 2 teaspoons cornstarch, tapioca starch, or arrowroot OR 1 tablespoon of
>   QuickThick™ or ThickenUp™
> ⅓ cup wine vinegar, apple cider vinegar, or lemon juice OR 1½ teaspoons
>   unbuffered vitamin C powder plus ⅓ cup water
> 2 teaspoons agave, Fruit Sweet™ or honey (optional)
> 1 tablespoon paprika
> 1 teaspoon salt
> Dash of pepper
> 1 cup oil, preferably walnut or canola because they are high in essential
>   fatty acids

If you are using the cornstarch, tapioca starch, or arrowroot, combine it with the ¼ cup of water in a saucepan. Cook the mixture over medium heat until it reaches the boiling point, becomes thick, and clears somewhat. Allow it to cool slightly. Put the cooked starch mixture or the ¼ cup water and QuickThick™ or

ThickenUp™ in a large measuring cup or the tall container that came with your hand blender. (You can use a standard blender or food processor instead). Add the vinegar, lemon juice, or vitamin C plus water, sweetener, paprika, salt, and pepper. Blend until thoroughly mixed. While you continue blending, add the oil gradually in a slow stream. Refrigerate the dressing until meal time or serve it immediately on salad. Refrigerate any leftover dressing. Makes about 1⅔ cups of dressing.

Lower fat variation: Use ¾ cup water in place of the ¼ cup water, 3 tablespoons of cornstarch, tapioca starch or arrowroot OR ¼ cup QuickThick™ or ThickenUp™, and ½ cup of oil.

Sweet Yogurt Dressing

Gluten-Free

1 cup GF plain yogurt (cow, goat, sheep, soy, or any other kind you
    tolerate)
2 tablespoons lemon juice or ¼ teaspoon unbuffered vitamin C powder
¼ cup apple or pineapple juice concentrate, thawed, or 2 tablespoons of
    agave, Fruit Sweet™ or honey
¼ teaspoon salt
1 teaspoon poppy seeds (optional)

If you are using the vitamin C, thoroughly stir it into a few tablespoons of the yogurt. Add the rest of the ingredients and thoroughly stir them together. Serve the dressing immediately or refrigerate it until meal time. Refrigerate any leftover dressing. Makes about 1⅓ cups of dressing.

Herbed Yogurt Dressing

Gluten-Free

1 cup GF plain yogurt (cow, goat, sheep, soy, or any other kind you
    tolerate)
2 tablespoons of lemon juice or ¼ teaspoon unbuffered vitamin C
    powder
⅛ to ¼ teaspoon pepper, or to taste
¼ teaspoon salt
1 teaspoon dry oregano or sweet basil

If you are using the vitamin C, thoroughly stir it into a few tablespoons of the yogurt. Add the rest of the ingredients and thoroughly stir them together. Serve the dressing immediately or refrigerate it until meal time. Refrigerate any leftover dressing. Makes about 1 cup of dressing.

Super-Smooth Sauce

Gluten-Free

This mayonnaise substitute is made from natural nut butters. It is a great source of essential fatty acids and a good replacement for mayonnaise for those who are allergic to eggs. If you are allergic to lemon or lime juice, use the vitamin C.

Cashew sauce

> ¼ cup cashew butter
> ¼ cup lemon or lime juice or ¼ cup water plus 1½ teaspoons unbuffered
>   vitamin C powder
> ⅛ teaspoon salt
> ¼ cup oil

Almond sauce

> ¼ cup almond butter
> ¼ cup lemon or lime juice or ¼ cup water plus 1 teaspoon unbuffered
>   vitamin C powder
> ⅛ teaspoon salt
> ¼ cup oil

Macadamia sauce

> ¼ cup macadamia nut butter
> ¼ cup lemon or lime juice or ¼ cup water plus 1 teaspoon unbuffered
>   vitamin C powder
> ⅛ teaspoon salt
> ¼ cup oil

Chose one set of ingredients from the list above. Combine the nut butter, lemon or lime juice or water plus vitamin C and salt in a 2-cup glass measuring cup or the tall narrow cup that came with your hand blender. Turn on the blender and blend until the ingredients are thoroughly combined. (You can use a standard blender or food processor instead). With the blender running, add the oil very gradually in a thin steam until it has all been added and the sauce is thick, smooth, and creamy. Makes about ¾ cup of sauce. Store in the refrigerator.

Mayonnaise

Gluten-Free

Here's real mayonnaise for those of you who can eat eggs. It is made without vinegar for those who are allergic to yeast. Although not exactly a "with ease" recipe, it is so delicious that it's well worth the small amount of extra time it takes to make it.

> 1 pasteurized egg or ¼ cup GF egg substitute such as EggBeaters™ (if you tolerate the ingredients)*
> 1 teaspoon dry ground mustard
> 1 teaspoon salt
> Dash of pepper
> 1 teaspoon agave, Fruit Sweet™ or honey (optional)
> 1 cup oil, divided, preferably walnut or canola because they are high in essential fatty acids
> 3 tablespoons lemon juice

Combine the egg or egg substitute, mustard, salt, pepper, sweetener, and ¼ cup of the oil in the bowl of a food processor or blender. Turn on the food processor or blender. After the ingredients are thoroughly mixed (this takes just a few seconds), very slowly, pouring in a trickle, add half of the remaining oil while processing continuously. At this point, you may stop processing. Add the lemon juice and begin processing again. After the lemon juice is mixed in (again, this takes just a few seconds), very slowly, pouring in a trickle, add the rest of the oil while processing continuously. Makes about 1½ cups of mayonnaise. Store in the refrigerator.

*Note: Pasteurized eggs are available in a few areas of the country and should be more widely available soon. If this mayonnaise will not be eaten by anyone in a high-risk population for serious illness due to *Salmonella* (the very young or the elderly), the USDA now says it is all right to use a regular raw egg in mayonnaise. EggBeaters™ and similar egg products are pasteurized, eliminating the problem of illness from using the egg raw, but they contain the egg white and other allergenic ingredients, some of which may be derived from wheat. At the time of this writing, EggBeaters™ is wheat- and gluten-free but contains maltodextrin which comes from corn.

Easy Side Dishes

Although they are not the main attraction, side dishes are economical, add a lot of nutrition to a meal, and also are usually easier to cook than main dishes. This chapter gives you recipes for side dishes such as stovetop-cooked grains and vegetables, spreads and dips. For other side dish recipes such as oven grains and vegetables, see pages 80 to 85. For side dishes cooked in the microwave, see pages 105 to 112.

Grains and Grain Alternatives

Stove Top Grains

Gluten-Free

If you wish to cook other grains such as kamut, amaranth, rye, oat groats, spelt, or barley on the stove, see pages 90-92 of The Ultimate Food Allergy Cookbook and Survival Guide *which is described on the last pages of this book.*

Brown rice
>   1 cup brown rice
>   2½ cups water
>   ¼ teaspoon salt
>   Cooking time: 45 to 50 minutes

White rice
>   1 cup white rice
>   2 cups water
>   ¼ teaspoon salt
>   Cooking time: 20 minutes

Wild rice
>   1 cup wild rice
>   4 cups water
>   ¼ teaspoon salt
>   Cooking time: 60 minutes

Quinoa
>   1 cup quinoa
>   2 cups water
>   ¼ teaspoon salt
>   Cooking time: 20 minutes

Teff

1 cup teff
3 cups water
¼ teaspoon salt
    Cooking time: 15 to 20 minutes

Millet

1 cup millet
3 cups water
¼ teaspoon salt
    Cooking time: 25 to 35 minutes

Sorghum (Milo)

1 cup sorghum (milo)
3½ cups water
¼ teaspoon salt
    Cooking time: 1 to 1¼ hours

Buckwheat, raw or white

1 cup buckwheat
3 cups water
½ teaspoon salt
    Cooking time: 20 to 25 minutes

Buckwheat, roasted

1 cup roasted buckwheat
2½ cups water
½ teaspoon salt
    Cooking time: 20 to 30 minutes

Choose one set of ingredients above. If you are cooking quinoa, be sure to rinse it in a strainer under running water until the water is no longer sudsy to remove its natural soapy coating.

For fluffy grains, put the water into a saucepan and bring it to a boil. Add the grain and salt. Put the lid on the pan and return it to a boil. Then lower the heat and simmer it for the time specified with the ingredient list for the grain you are cooking. Remove the pan from the heat. Allow the grain to stand for a few minutes, fluff it with a fork, and serve.

For creamy rather than fluffy grains, combine the grain, water, and salt in a saucepan. Put the lid on the pan. Bring it to a boil; then lower the heat and simmer it for the time specified with the ingredient list. Remove the pan from the heat. Allow the grain to stand for a few minutes before serving.

Makes about 2 cups of cooked grain or 4 servings.

Savory Celery Grain Pilaf

Gluten-Free

Although this recipe has a few more ingredients than others in this chapter, it is still quick to make and is a nice change from plain grains.

> 2 cups sliced celery
> ¼ small onion, chopped or 1 tablespoon dry chopped onions (optional)
> 4 tablespoons oil
> 1 cup of any grain from the "Stove Top Grains" recipe, pages 126 to 127
> Water in the amount specified for the chosen grain in the "Stove Top
>   Grains" recipe, pages 126 to127
> ½ to 1 teaspoon salt, to taste
> ¼ teaspoon black pepper
> 1 tablespoon dried parsley
> 1 teaspoon dried sweet basil

Combine the celery, fresh onion (if you are using it), and oil in a saucepan. Place it on the stove over medium heat and cook it until the vegetables begin to brown. Add the grain, optional dry onion, and water to the pan. Bring the pan to a boil over medium to high heat. Reduce the heat and simmer it for the time specified for the grain you are using in the "Stove Top Grains" recipe, pages 126 to 127. Stir the pepper, parsley, and sweet basil into the grain. Remove the pan from the heat and allow it to stand for a few minutes before serving. Makes 6 to 9 servings.

Sweet and Spicy Rice

Gluten-Free

When you make this, you will spend a little more time than usual chopping celery and measuring seasonings, but this is a change from plain grains that everyone really enjoys.

> 2 tablespoons oil
> ¼ cup chopped onion or 1 tablespoon dry chopped onions (optional)
> ¾ cup sliced celery
> 1 to 1½ teaspoons salt, to taste
> ¼ teaspoon pepper
> ¼ teaspoon cinnamon
> ⅛ teaspoon allspice
> 1 cup white rice
> ½ cup plus 1 tablespoon apple juice concentrate, thawed

2 to 2½ cups water
½ cup raisins
⅓ cup chopped or slivered almonds (optional)

Combine the oil, celery, and fresh onion, if you are using it, in a saucepan. Cook them over medium heat until the vegetables are just beginning to become tender. Add the optional dry onions, salt, pepper, cinnamon, allspice, rice, apple juice concentrate, 2 cups of the water, and raisins. Put the cover on the pan. Bring it to a boil over medium to medium-high heat. Reduce the heat and simmer for 25 to 30 minutes or until all the liquid is absorbed and the rice is tender. Check the rice occasionally during the last ten minutes of cooking to see if the liquid has been absorbed. If so and the rice is not tender yet, you may have had extra-dry raisins and will need to add another ½ cup of water and cook the rice for another 5 to 10 minutes or until the liquid is all absorbed. When the rice is tender, remove it from the heat and let it stand 5 minutes. Fluff the rice with a fork and stir in the nuts. Let it stand a few more minutes before serving. Makes 6 to 9 servings.

Vegetables

The most easily cooked and often most economical vegetables come from the freezer section of your grocery store. Read their bags for instructions because how long you cook them will vary from brand to brand depending on the processing the vegetables received before freezing. However, there are some fresh vegetables that you may want to prepare, especially when they are in season and on sale, so recipes are included for them here. Be sure to notice "Oven Fries" which are a quick, nutritious take-off on French fries.

Instructions are given in this chapter for cooking a few commonly eaten and easily prepared fresh vegetables on the stove top. This section does not include vegetables such as corn cut from the cob, beans and peas because if you are short on time, you will want to use frozen corn, beans, and peas rather than shelling, stringing, cutting, and shucking fresh vegetables. To cook less commonly eaten fresh vegetables, see the "Vegetable Primer" chapter in *Easy Cooking for Special Diets* as described on the last pages of this book.

Although steaming is the ideal way to cook vegetables on the stove top for preserving nutrients, a steamer is another piece of cooking equipment that will have to be washed after the meal! Therefore, I usually cook vegetables on the stove top in a *small* amount of water. That way most of the vegetables are above the water and are actually being steamed, and the nutrients are better preserved than if you boil the vegetables in copious amounts of water.

Oven Fries

Gluten-Free

Have fries without much fat! You can cook these in the oven while you are preparing an entrée on the stove top and making a salad.

> 1 pound of white potatoes
> 1 tablespoon oil (optional)
> ¼ teaspoon salt

Preheat your oven on to 425°F. Scrub or peel the potatoes and cut them into ⅓ to ½ inch sticks or fries. Put them on a non-stick baking sheet, drizzle with the oil, and sprinkle them with the salt. Mix the potatoes with your hand so that all sides of the fries are coated with oil. Spread them out in a single layer on the baking sheet. (You can use a regular baking sheet but you may wish to use slightly more oil to make them easier to turn). Bake for 15 to 20 minutes or until they begin to brown on the bottom. Turn them with a spatula and bake for another 15 minutes or until they are brown. If they take much longer than 30 minutes to cook, turn the oven temperature up to 450°F the next time you make these fries. Makes 3 to 4 servings.

Mashed Potatoes

Gluten-Free

Yes, you CAN make mashed potatoes without dairy products! Mashed potatoes take a little time, but they are delicious even when milk-free. Use a thin-skinned potato variety such as Yukon Gold and scrub rather than peel the potatoes. You will save time and also benefit from the vitamins and minerals that are found right under the skin.

> 6 medium sized potatoes, or about 2 pounds of potatoes of any size
> 4 cups water
> 1 to 1½ teaspoons salt, divided, or to taste
> 3 tablespoons of oil, Earth Balance™ margarine, butter or goat butter
> ⅓ cup water, skim, whole, goat, or other alternative milk

Wash and peel or scrub the potatoes. Cut the potatoes into quarters, or to save time, into smaller cubes which will cook more quickly. Put them in a saucepan with the 4 cups of water and ½ teaspoon of the salt and cover the pan. Bring them to a boil over medium heat. Reduce the heat and simmer them for 20 to 45 minutes, or until they are tender when pierced with a fork. Pour off the water. Reserve ⅓ cup of the cooking water if you are not going to use milk. Add the reserved water or milk, oil, margarine or butter, and ½ teaspoon of salt to the pan and mash the potatoes with a potato masher. Taste them and add the remaining ½ teaspoon salt if needed. If they seem dry, add more milk or water. Mash in the additional salt and liquid if you added them. If you are allergic to milk including alternative milk, use water or reserved potato cooking water instead of milk and use oil or milk- and trans-fat-free Earth Balance™ margarine instead of butter. Makes about 6 servings.

Asparagus

Gluten-Free

Hold both ends of each asparagus stalk and bend. Discard the root end. Swish the stalks in a sink of cold water, allowing a little soaking time to loosen any dirt that might be hiding in the tips. If there is any dirt or grit in the bottom of the sink, change the water and swish again until the grit is all removed. Take the asparagus from the water.

Put the asparagus in a pan with water and bring it to a boil. Simmer until it is done to your preference. To cook it to tenderness will take 10 to 15 minutes. Drain and serve with butter or oil and salt.

Broccoli

Gluten-Free

Trim off any leaves and cut the stems to about 4 inches in length. Wash the broccoli and cut it into spears by cutting downward between the stalks.

Bring about ½ inch of water to boil in a saucepan. Add the broccoli, return the water to a boil and simmer until the broccoli is tender, about 10 to 15 minutes, or until it is done to your preference. Serve with a little butter or oil and salt and/or pepper if desired.

Cabbage

Gluten-Free

Cut a head of cabbage into wedges or core it and chop or shred it. In a sauce-pan, heat one inch of water and ½ teaspoon of salt to the boiling point. Add the cabbage. Cover and bring the water back to a boil. Lower the heat and simmer cabbage wedges about 15 minutes for green cabbage or 20 minutes for red cabbage. Simmer chopped or shredded cabbage about 5 to 10 minutes, or until it is done to your preference. Drain and serve with oil and salt if desired.

Cauliflower

Gluten-Free

Wash the cauliflower and remove the outer leaves. Cut off any dark spots from the florets. Cut the florets from the center core. In a saucepan, heat one inch of water and ½ teaspoon of salt to the boiling point. Add the cauliflower. Cover and bring the water back to a boil. Lower the heat and simmer about 10 to 13 minutes, or until the cauliflower is done to your preference. Drain and serve with butter or oil and salt if desired.

Corn on the Cob

Gluten-Free

Remove the husks from fresh corn. Break or cut off the stem end. Remove any tassel strings that cling to the corn by wiping the ear with a damp piece of paper towel from the narrow tip of the ear to the end where the husk was attached. Bring a large pot of water to a boil. Add the corn. Return the water to a boil and cook for two to five minutes. Drain and serve.

Spinach and Other Greens

Gluten-Free

If you do not like frozen spinach, used the pre-washed bagged spinach that is sold with the salad greens. This recipe can also be used for other greens such as collards, kale, chard, etc. If you use young (baby) spinach, you do not need to remove the stems.

Remove the stem ends from the spinach or greens. Put the leaves in a sink filled with cool water and swish them around. Lift them out into the other side of the sink, fill the sink with water, and swish them again. Repeat this several times until there is no more dirt left in the water when you lift the greens out. If you are using pre-washed spinach, it (obviously) does not need to be washed. Just put it in the sink with water to get it wet before proceeding with this recipe.

Put the leaves into a large pan with the water still clinging to the leaves. Heat over medium heat, stirring occasionally, until they come to a boil. Reduce the heat and cook for 5 to 10 minutes or until they are done to your preference. Serve with butter or oil and salt if desired.

Spreads and Dips

Garbanzo Dip

Gluten-Free

Although these spreads and dips are more appetizers than side dishes, they are good to have with a meal as an accompaniment for fresh vegetable crudités or a healthy variety of chips.

> 1 16-ounce can of garbanzo beans, drained, or about 1½ to 1¾ cup of beans
> ⅓ cup water
> ¼ to ½ teaspoon salt, or to taste
> 2 teaspoons tart-tasting unbuffered vitamin C powder
> ⅛ teaspoon dry mustard (optional)
> ⅛ teaspoon pepper (optional)

Put the beans in a blender or food processor with the metal pureeing blade. Process them using a pulsing action until they are finely ground. Add all of the other ingredients and puree until smooth. (You may have to do this in small batches if you are using a blender). Refrigerate the dip. Serve spread on crackers or rice cakes or use it as a dip for raw vegetables. You can freeze any leftover dip in serving-sized portions. Makes about 2 cups of dip.

Lentil Spread

Gluten-Free

Serve this spread with raw vegetables as a dip, on crackers, or in sandwiches. It tastes somewhat like liverwurst or paté.

> 1 15-ounce can* of lentils, drained, or about 1½ cups of cooked lentils
> ½ to 1 onion, peeled and chopped or 2 to 3 tablespoons dry chopped
>   onions (optional, but the onion gives the spread most of its flavor)
> 1 tablespoon oil (only needed if using fresh onion)
> ½ cup walnuts or other nuts or ¼ cup mild-tasting natural nut butter
> 1 to 1¼ teaspoons salt
> ½ teaspoon pepper, or more to taste

If using the fresh onion, sauté it in the oil until it is soft, or soak the dry onion in hot water for a few minutes until rehydrated and then drain off the excess water. Grind the walnuts with the pureeing blade of a food processor. (If you with to use a blender or hand-blender, you will have to make this recipe with nut butter. Since this mixture is thick, it is worth getting out the processor if you have one). Add the rest of the ingredients to the ground nuts or nut butter and puree until smooth. Taste and adjust the seasonings. Refrigerate the spread or freeze it in serving-sized portions. Makes about 2 to 2½ cups of spread

Note: Canned lentils can be difficult to find. Your health food store may carry Westbrae™ Organic Lentils which contain just lentils, water, and sea salt.

Cottage Cheese Dip

Gluten-Free

1 carrot
3 large radishes
1 cup low-fat cottage cheese
¼ cup plain low-fat yogurt, sour cream, or mayonnaise
½ teaspoon salt
¼ teaspoon pepper
2 teaspoons caraway seeds (optional)

Peel the carrot and grate it by rubbing it over the largest holes of a cheese grater. Finely chop the radishes. Put the cottage cheese in a bowl and puree it with a hand blender, food processor or standard blender until smooth. Add the yogurt, sour cream or mayonnaise, salt, and pepper and puree the dip again briefly. Stir in the caraway seeds, carrot, and radishes. Refrigerate until serving time. Makes about 1¾ cups of dip or 7 servings.

Guacamole

Gluten-Free

1 large ripe avocado, weighing about ½ pound
1½ teaspoons lemon juice or ⅛ teaspoon unbuffered vitamin C powder
1 tablespoon finely chopped onion or 1 teaspoon dry onion (optional)
1 green chili pepper, finely chopped (optional)
1 small tomato, peeled and finely chopped (optional)
¼ teaspoon salt, or to taste
⅛ to ¼ teaspoon pepper, to taste (optional)

Peel and seed the avocado. Put it in a bowl with the lemon juice or vitamin C, onion, chili pepper, salt, and pepper. Mash all of the ingredients together thoroughly with a fork or blend them with a hand blender. Gently fold in the tomato. Serve the dip immediately. This sauce may darken if it stands very long. Makes about ⅔ to 1 cup of dip or 6 servings.

Muffins, Crackers and Bread

Bread and similar foods are the staff of life. Because complex carbohydrates are an ideal energy source, whole-grain breads are important part of our diets. Grain-based foods also provide essential nutrients such as fiber, vitamins, and minerals. Without bread – or something like it – a meal does not seem complete and our nutrition may be less than optimal. However, routinely using commercially made baked goods can be expensive. Baking at home not only saves money but will also help you preserve tolerance to rice for those times when you eat out or can't bake.

Celiacs may be able to purchase bread and crackers that they can eat pre-made, but those with multiple food allergies who need to rotate their foods will have to bake some of these foods for themselves. Everyone, whether on a special diet or not, enjoys a freshly baked treat occasionally. Using these recipes you can make nutritious goodies for your special diet quickly and easily.

Amaranth Blueberry Muffins

Gluten-Free

If you can't finish eating a whole batch of these muffins within a day or so, freeze them to maintain their moistness.

1¾ cups amaranth flour
½ cup arrowroot
2 teaspoons baking soda
½ teaspoon unbuffered vitamin C powder
¼ teaspoon cloves (optional)
¾ cup apple juice concentrate, thawed,
¼ cup oil
¾ cup dried blueberries* or moist raisins (optional)

Preheat your oven to 375°F. Line 12 wells of a muffin pan with paper muffin cup liners. Mix the amaranth flour, arrowroot, baking soda, and vitamin C powder in a large bowl. Stir in the dried fruit. Stir together the apple juice and oil. Pour the liquid ingredients into the dry ingredients and stir until they are just mixed. The batter will be stiffer than for most muffins. Put the batter into the prepared muffin tin filling the cups about ⅞ full. Bake for 15 to 20 minutes or until the muffins brown and a toothpick inserted in the center comes out dry. Makes 10 to 12 muffins.

*Note: To make these muffins with fresh or frozen blueberries (which is just slightly more work), see page 140.

Oatmeal Muffins

Ask your doctor.

Oats are tolerated by some celiacs but not others. Ask your doctor if you should eat oats before trying these muffins.

    2 cups oat flour
    ¼ teaspoon salt (optional)
    1 teaspoon baking soda
    ¼ teaspoon unbuffered vitamin C powder
    ¼ cup oil
    1 cup water

Preheat your oven to 400°F. Line 10 wells of a muffin pan with paper liners or oil and flour them with oat flour. Mix the flour, salt, baking soda, and vitamin C powder together in a large bowl. Mix together the water and oil, pour them into the dry ingredients, and stir until they are just mixed in. Put the batter into the prepared muffin tin, filling the cups about ⅔ full. Bake for 30 to 35 minutes, or until the muffins begin to brown and pull away from the side of the pan. Makes about 10 muffins.

Barley Muffins

These are delicious for breakfast and are great with soup for dinner.

    2 cups barley flour
    ¼ teaspoon salt (optional)
    1 teaspoon baking soda
    ¼ teaspoon unbuffered vitamin C powder
    ¼ cup oil
    1¼ cups water or apple juice

Preheat your oven to 400°F. Line 12 wells of a muffin pan with paper liners or oil and flour them with barley flour. Mix the flour, salt, baking soda, and vitamin C powder in a large bowl. Stir optional variety* ingredients (see below) into the flour mixture. Mix the juice or water with the oil, pour them into the dry ingredients, and stir until they are just mixed in. Fill the muffin cups about ⅔ full. Bake for 30 to 35 minutes or until the muffins begin to brown and a toothpick inserted into the center comes out dry. Makes about 12 muffins

*Note: For variety, add ⅔ cup of raisins or other diced dry fruit or nuts and/or 1 teaspoon of cinnamon to the muffins.

Pineapple Muffins

Gluten-Free IF
made with sorghum or teff

Delicately flavorful, these muffins are a hit with young and old alike especially when made with sorghum flour.

2 cups sorghum (milo) flour OR 2 cups teff flour OR 2¼ cups spelt flour
1 teaspoon baking soda
¼ teaspoon unbuffered vitamin C powder
½ cup pineapple canned in juice or fresh pineapple with juice to cover
½ cup pineapple juice concentrate, thawed
⅓ cup oil

Puree the pineapple and its juice with a hand blender, standard blender, or food processor. Preheat your oven to 400°F. Line 12 wells of a muffin pan with paper liners or oil and flour them with the flour you are using in the recipe. Mix the flour, baking soda, and vitamin C powder in a large bowl. Combine the pureed pineapple, pineapple juice concentrate, and oil and stir them into the dry ingredients until they are just mixed in. Put the batter into the prepared muffin tin, filling the cups about ⅔ full. Bake for 15 to 20 minutes or until the muffins begin to brown. Makes about 12 muffins.

Apple and Spice Muffins

Gluten-Free

The chunks of apple or raisins add a sweet surprise to these spicy grain-free muffins.

1¾ cups quinoa flour
¼ cup tapioca flour
2 teaspoons baking soda
½ teaspoon unbuffered vitamin C powder
2 teaspoons cinnamon
1¼ cups peeled and chopped apples or ¾ cup moist raisins (optional)
1 cup unsweetened applesauce
¼ cup apple juice concentrate, thawed
¼ cup oil

Preheat your oven to 375°F. Line 16 wells of a muffin pan with paper liners or oil and flour them with quinoa flour. Mix the flours, baking soda, vitamin C powder and cinnamon together. Stir the chopped apples or raisins into the dry ingredients. Mix together the applesauce, apple juice and oil, and add them to the dry ingredients, stirring until just mixed. Put the batter into an oiled and floured muffin tin, filling the muffin cups about ¾ full. Bake for 20 to 25 minutes or until the muffins brown and a toothpick inserted in the center comes out dry. Makes about 16 muffins.

Spelt Muffins

These muffins have a delicious whole-grain nutty flavor.

2½ cups spelt flour
1½ teaspoons baking soda
¼ teaspoon unbuffered vitamin C powder
⅓ cup oil
1 cup apple juice concentrate, thawed

Preheat your oven to 350°F. Line 12 wells of a muffin pan with paper liners or oil and flour them with spelt flour. Mix the flour, baking soda, and vitamin C powder in a large bowl. Stir optional variety* ingredients (see below) into the flour mixture. Mix the juice with the oil, pour them into the dry ingredients, and stir until just mixed. Fill the muffin cups about ⅔ full. Bake for 15 to 18 minutes or until the muffins begin to brown and a toothpick inserted into the center comes out dry. Makes about 12 muffins.

*Note: For variety, add ⅔ cup of raisins or other diced dry fruit or nuts and/or 1 teaspoon of cinnamon to the muffins.

Kamut Muffins

These are great with blueberries! See the "Blueberry Muffins" recipe on page 140.

2¼ cups kamut flour
1½ teaspoon baking soda
¼ teaspoon unbuffered vitamin C powder
¼ cup oil
1¼ cups apple juice concentrate, thawed

Preheat your oven to 350°F. Line 11 wells of a muffin pan with paper liners or oil and flour them with kamut flour. Mix the flour, baking soda, and vitamin C powder in a large bowl. Stir optional variety* ingredients (see below) into the flour mixture. Mix the juice with the oil, pour them into the dry ingredients, and stir until just mixed. Fill the muffin cups about ⅔ full. Bake for 25 to 30 minutes or until the muffins begin to brown and a toothpick inserted into the center comes out dry. Makes 10 to 11 muffins.

*Note: For variety, add ⅔ cup of raisins or other diced dry fruit or nuts and/or 1 teaspoon of cinnamon to the muffins.

Rye Muffins

> 2 cups rye flour
> ¾ teaspoon baking soda
> ¼ teaspoon unbuffered vitamin C powder if water and maple syrup are used; ⅛ teaspoon if juice is used
> ⅓ cup oil
> 1 cup unsweetened white grape juice or apple juice OR ⅓ cup maple syrup plus ⅔ cup water

Preheat your oven to 400°F. Line 12 wells of a muffin pan with paper liners or oil and flour them with rye flour. Mix the flour, baking soda, and vitamin C powder in a large bowl. Stir optional variety* ingredients (see below) into the flour mixture. Mix the juice or maple syrup plus water with the oil, pour them into the dry ingredients, and stir until just mixed. Fill the muffin cups about ⅔ full. Bake for 18 to 20 minutes or until the muffins begin to brown and a toothpick inserted into the center comes out dry. Makes about 12 muffins.

*Note: For variety, add ⅔ cup of raisins or other diced dry fruit or nuts and/or 1 teaspoon of cinnamon to the muffins.

Fresh or Frozen Blueberry Muffins

**Gluten-Free IF
made with amaranth**

With just a few moments of extra time, you can make the muffin recipes on the preceding pages deliciously special.

> 1 cup fresh blueberries or unsweetened frozen blueberries, not thawed
> 1 batch of one of the following recipes:
>> Amaranth Blueberry Muffins, page 135
>> Oatmeal Muffins, page 135
>> Barley Muffins, page 136
>> Spelt Muffins page 138
>> Kamut Muffins, page 138
>> Rye Muffins page 139

If you are using frozen blueberries, put them in a strainer and rinse them with cold running water just until the water is no longer highly purple. Preheat your oven to the temperature specified in the recipe. Mix the muffin batter as directed in the recipe omitting dried blueberries or other dried fruit. Quickly fold in the fresh or frozen blueberries. Bake as directed in the recipe with fresh blueberries or for 5 to 10 minutes longer if you are using frozen blueberries. Makes one or two more muffins than what the recipe would make without the blueberries.

Quinoa Sesame Seed Crackers

Gluten-Free

These crackers make a delicious snack that will satisfy your hunger and stick with you for a long time.

> 3 cups quinoa flour
> 1 cup tapioca starch
> ⅓ cup sesame seeds
> 5¼ teaspoons GF baking powder OR 2 teaspoons baking soda plus ½
>> teaspoon unbuffered vitamin C powder
> 1 teaspoon salt
> 1¼ cups water
> ½ cup oil

Preheat your oven to 350°F. Mix together the quinoa flour, tapioca starch, sesame seeds, baking powder or baking soda plus vitamin C powder, and salt in a large bowl. Combine the water and oil and stir them into the dry ingredients until the dough comes together. Divide the dough into thirds. Roll each third to about ⅛ inch thickness on an ungreased baking sheet using an oiled rolling pin. If the dough sticks to the rolling pin, lightly flour the top of the dough. After rolling, cut the dough into 2-inch squares and sprinkle the tops of the crackers with salt if desired. Bake for 15 to 25 minutes, or until the crackers are crisp and lightly browned. If the crackers around the edges of the baking sheet brown before the center, remove them from the baking sheet and allow the crackers in the center to bake longer. Cool the crackers on paper towels. Makes about 9 dozen crackers.

Amaranth Crackers

Gluten-Free

These crackers are so good that I would like to eat them every day.

3 cups amaranth flour
1 cup arrowroot
2 teaspoons baking soda
½ teaspoon unbuffered vitamin C powder
1 teaspoon salt
¾ cup water
½ cup oil

Preheat your oven to 375°F. Combine the amaranth flour, arrowroot, baking soda, vitamin C powder, and salt in a large bowl. Mix together the water and oil and pour them into the flour mixture. Stir until the dough sticks together, adding another few tablespoons of water if necessary to form a stiff but not crumbly dough. Divide the dough into thirds. Roll each third to about ⅛ inch thickness on an ungreased baking sheet and cut the dough into 2 inch squares. Sprinkle the tops of the crackers lightly with additional salt if desired. Bake for 15 to 20 minutes, or until the crackers are crisp and lightly browned. If the crackers around the edges of the baking sheet brown before the center, remove them from the baking sheet and allow the crackers in the center to bake longer. Cool the crackers on paper towels. Makes about 9 dozen crackers.

Oat Crackers

Ask your doctor.

These crackers are tasty and easy to make with just four ingredients.

    4 cups quick oats, uncooked
    ½ teaspoon salt
    ⅓ cup oil
    ⅔ cup water

Preheat your oven to 350°F. Lightly oil two baking sheets. Stir the oats and salt together. Add the oil and mix it into the dry ingredients thoroughly. Stir in the water, then mix and knead the dough with your hands until it sticks together. Divide the dough in half; put each half on one of the prepared baking sheets. Lightly rub your rolling pin with oil. Roll the cracker dough out to about ⅛ inch thickness. Cut the dough into 1½ inch squares and sprinkle the crackers lightly with salt. Bake the crackers for 20 to 25 minutes. Watch the crackers closely as the baking time nears completion. If the crackers on the edges of the sheets brown before the baking time is up, remove them from the baking sheet and continue to bake the rest of the crackers. Use a spatula to remove the crackers from the baking sheets when they begin to brown. Put them on paper towels to cool. Makes 3 to 4 dozen crackers.

Quinoa "Graham" Crackers

Gluten-Free

My friend and taster Athena really likes these grain-free "graham" crackers.

    3 cups quinoa flour
    1 cup tapioca starch
    3 teaspoons GF baking powder plus ½ teaspoon baking soda OR 2
        teaspoons baking soda plus ½ teaspoon unbuffered vitamin C powder
    ½ teaspoon cinnamon (optional)
    1¼ cups apple juice concentrate
    ½ cup oil

Preheat your oven to 350°F. Oil three baking sheets. Mix together the quinoa flour, tapioca starch, baking powder (if you are using it), baking soda, vitamin C powder (if you are using them), and cinnamon in a large bowl. Combine the apple juice concentrate and oil and stir them into the dry ingredients until the dough sticks together. Divide the dough into thirds and put each third on one of the baking sheets. Flour your rolling pin and the top of the dough. Roll each third to just under ¼ inch thickness. Flour a knife and cut the dough into 1 inch by 3 inch bars. You may have to re-flour the knife between cuts. Prick each bar three times with a fork to resemble graham crackers. Bake for 10 to 15 minutes or until the crackers are lightly browned. Re-cut the crackers on the same lines if necessary. Remove the crackers from the baking sheet using a spatula, and allow them to cool on paper towels. Makes about 3 to 4 dozen crackers.

Spelt "Graham" Crackers

These fruit, agave, or honey-sweetened crackers are just like the ones you remember from your childhood.

      2⅝ cups whole spelt flour
      ½ teaspoon salt
      ¾ teaspoon baking soda
      ¼ teaspoon unbuffered vitamin C powder
      ½ teaspoon cinnamon (optional)
      ½ cup oil
      ½ cup agave or Fruit Sweet™ or agave OR ⅜ cup honey plus ⅛ cup water

Preheat your oven to 350°F. Lightly oil two baking sheets and dust them with spelt flour. Combine the flour, salt, baking soda, vitamin C powder, and cinnamon in a large bowl. Thoroughly mix together the oil with the Fruit Sweet™ or agave or the honey and water until the mixture looks granular. Immediately stir the liquids into the flour mixture to form a soft dough. Divide the dough in half and put each portion of the dough on a prepared baking sheet. Sprinkle flour on top of the dough and rolling pin and roll each portion of dough to about ⅛ to just under ¼ inch thickness. Cut the dough into 1-inch by 3-inch rectangles and prick them with a fork. Bake for 12 to 17 minutes, or until they begin to brown. Remove them from the oven and re-cut them on the original cut lines if necessary. Remove them from the baking sheet with a spatula and cool them on paper towels. Makes 2½ to 4 dozen crackers.

Spelt Saltines

2 cups spelt flour
½ teaspoon salt
½ teaspoon baking soda
¼ teaspoon unbuffered vitamin C powder
¼ cup oil
½ cup water

Combine the flour, salt, baking soda, and vitamin C powder. Add the oil and stir until it is thoroughly mixed in to form small crumbs. Add the water two tablespoons at a time, mixing well after each addition. Knead the dough on a lightly floured board for one to two minutes. Divide the dough in half and roll each half out on an oiled baking sheet with an oiled rolling pin to about a 10 inch by 14 inch rectangle. The dough should be very thin, about ¹⁄₁₆ to ⅛ inch thick. Cut the dough into 2 inch squares and prick each square three times with a fork. Sprinkle the tops of the crackers with additional salt if desired. Bake at 350°F for 10 to 14 minutes, or until the crackers are golden brown and crisp. Cool the crackers on paper towels. Makes 6 to 7 dozen crackers.

Cassava Crackers

Gluten-Free

These delicious crackers are crunchy but crumbly. Save the crumbs to use in place of croutons in salads. To obtain cassava meal by mail order, see "Sources," page 209.

2 cups cassava meal
½ teaspoon baking soda
¼ teaspoon unbuffered vitamin C powder
¼ teaspoon salt
¾ cup water
¼ cup oil

Preheat your oven to 350°F. Oil a 12 by 15 inch pan. Mix the cassava meal, baking soda, vitamin C powder and salt together in a large bowl. Combine the water and oil and stir them into the dry ingredients. Roll and press the crumbly mixture firmly into the baking pan. (The thickness of the dough layer will be between ⅛ and ¼ inch). Cut the dough into 1½ inch squares and bake for 35 to 40 minutes. Remove the crackers from the pan with a spatula and cool them on paper towels. Makes about 3½ dozen crackers.

Cornbread

Gluten-Free

Cornmeal gives this bread a delightful crunchy texture.

¼ cup honey, agave, or Fruit Sweet™
¼ cup water (or you can use milk)
2 tablespoons oil
2 large eggs, slightly beaten
1 cup cornmeal
¼ teaspoon salt
2 teaspoons GF baking powder

Preheat your oven to 425°F. Oil an 8 by 4 inch or 9 by 5 inch loaf pan and shake cornmeal around the inside of the pan to coat it well. Stir together the sweetener and milk or water until the liquids are thoroughly mixed together. Add the oil and eggs and mix well. In a separate bowl, mix together the cornmeal, salt, and baking powder. Stir the liquid into the dry ingredients quickly and pour the batter into the prepared pan. Pop the cornbread into the oven. Bake for 20 to 25 minutes or until it is golden brown and a toothpick inserted in the center of the loaf comes out dry. Cool completely in the pan and then cut into squares to serve. Makes 6 to 8 servings.

Banana Bread

Gluten-Free IF
made with amaranth

This sweet and moist bread can be made in either gluten-free non-grain (amaranth) or grain-containing versions.

3 cups spelt flour OR 2½ cups barley flour OR 2 cups amaranth flour
     (GF) plus ½ cup arrowroot (GF)
½ teaspoon salt
2 teaspoons baking soda
½ teaspoon unbuffered vitamin C powder
½ teaspoon ground cloves or 1 teaspoon cinnamon (optional)
½ cup chopped nuts (optional)
1¾ cups thoroughly mashed or pureed ripe bananas
¼ cup oil

Preheat your oven to 350°F. Oil and flour (using the same flour you are baking with) a 9 by 5 inch loaf pan. Stir together the flour(s), baking soda, vitamin C powder, spice, salt, and nuts in a large bowl. Combine the mashed bananas and oil and stir them into the dry ingredients until they are completely mixed in, but be careful not to over-mix. (The batter will be stiff). Scrape the batter into the prepared loaf pan and bake for 55 to 60 minutes, or until the bread is lightly browned and a toothpick inserted in the center comes out dry. Remove it from the oven and allow it to cool in the pan for 10 minutes. Remove it from the pan to cool completely. Makes one loaf.

About Yeast Bread

The best way to make yeast bread "with ease" is to use an appliance such as a heavy duty mixer or a bread machine. Therefore, instructions for making bread totally by hand are not included in this chapter. If you have made yeast bread by hand, you can use the ingredient list for the gluten-containing spelt bread recipe on page 150 to make it the traditional way. The two gluten-free recipes below must be made by the mixer method or with a bread machine to develop the structure of the guar or xanthum gum.

For information about making bread by hand, see *Allergy Cooking With Ease* or *The Ultimate Food Allergy Cookbook and Survival Guide* which are described at the end of this book. For information on how to make yeast bread by hand, mixer, or bread machine and how to choose the bread machine that will work best for your special diet, see *Easy Breadmaking for Special Diets* as described on the last pages of this book.

If you already have a bread machine, you may be able to use it for special breads. Almost any machine can be used on the dough cycle to perform the initial mixing and kneading and the first rise for your bread. Then restart the cycle and allow the dough to knead for another 3 to 5 minutes. Remove the dough from the machine and put it in a prepared loaf pan. Proceed with the second rise and baking as in the following recipes.

Most gluten-free bread recipes are made with a combination of grains plus multiple stabilizers. This seems to produce bread with a more conventional texture in most cases. However, as you have read on previous pages, this book takes a different approach to combining several grains in each recipe both to save time on measuring and, more importantly, to prevent the development of allergies to foods that are eaten every day. Therefore, most of the recipes in this book are made with a single grain/grain alternative or a single grain/grain alternative plus a starch which acts as a binder. My two favorite single-grain gluten-free bread recipes are included in this chapter. For more bread recipes, both made by hand and by bread machine, see the books mentioned above.

Quinoa Raisin Yeast Bread

Gluten-Free

This tasty bread has an amazingly wheat-like texture for a gluten-free loaf. Try it toasted for breakfast.

> ¼ cup water
> ⅓ cup apple juice concentrate
> About 4 large or 3 extra large eggs* (enough to measure ¾ cup in
>   volume) at room temperature
> 2 tablespoons oil
> ¾ teaspoon salt
> 1 teaspoon cinnamon
> 4 teaspoons guar or xanthum gum*
> 2½ cups quinoa flour
> ¾ cup tapioca starch
> 2¼ teaspoons (1 package) GF active dry yeast
> ½ cup raisins

If you wish to use a bread machine to mix this bread, use the method described in the fourth paragraph on the previous page. After the first rise, start the cycle again and re-mix the dough for a few minutes. Add the raisins and mix for a minute or two more until they are evenly distributed in the dough. Proceed with this recipe as in the third paragraph of these directions.

To make this bread with a mixer, heat the water and apple juice concentrate to about 115°F. Beat the eggs slightly and measure ¾ cup. Stir together the dry ingredients in a large electric mixer bowl. With the mixer running at low speed, gradually add the liquid mixture, eggs, and oil. Beat the dough for three minutes at medium speed. Scrape the dough from the beaters and the sides of the bowl into the bottom of the bowl. Oil the top of the dough and the sides of the bowl, and cover the bowl with a towel. Put the bowl in a warm (85°F to 90°F) place* and let the dough rise for 1 to 1½ hours. Beat the dough again for three minutes at medium speed. Stir in the raisins by hand.

Oil and flour an 8 by 4 inch loaf pan. Put the dough in the pan and allow it to rise in a warm place for about 20 to 30 minutes or until it barely doubles. Preheat the oven to 375°F. Bake the loaf for about 50 to 70 minutes, loosely covering it with foil after the first 15 minutes to prevent excessive browning. Remove the loaf from the pan and cool it completely on a cooling rack. Makes one loaf.

*Notes: If you are allergic to eggs, use ¾ cup warm water in their place. If you do not take the eggs out of the refrigerator early enough for them to come to room temperature before you are ready to bake, put them in a bowl of warm water for 5 or 10 minutes before cracking them to use in this recipe.

On guar or xanthum gum: When making the dough for this bread in a bread machine, mix together the guar or xanthum gum and flour before adding them to the machine. If you just add the ingredients to the machine in the order listed, during the warm-up time before mixing begins, the water and gum can form lumps that routine mixing may not completely eliminate.

On a warm rising place: To use your oven as a cozy place for bread to rise, see the third paragraph on page 179.

Buckwheat "Rye" Bread

Gluten-Free

The caraway seeds and rye flavor powder give this bread a delicious rye-like taste. If you are a rye fan like I am, watch out! I have to freeze part of the loaf to keep from finishing the whole thing in two days. If you do not like rye, this bread is also delicious without the rye flavor.

½ cup water
¼ cup apple juice concentrate
About 4 large or 3 extra large eggs*, or enough to measure ¾ cup in
    volume, at room temperature
3 tablespoons oil
1¼ teaspoon salt
1 tablespoon caraway seed (optional)
¾ teaspoon rye flavor powder, to taste (optional; see "Sources," page 211)
1 tablespoon guar or xanthum gum*
2 cups buckwheat flour
1⅜ cup tapioca starch
2¼ teaspoons (1 package) GF active dry yeast

If you wish to use a bread machine to mix this bread, use the method described in the fourth paragraph on page 146. After the first rise, re-start the cycle and re-mix the dough for a few minutes. Then proceed with this recipe as in the third paragraph of these directions.

To make this bread using a mixer, heat the water and apple juice concentrate to about 115°F. Beat the eggs slightly and add them to the other liquids. Stir together the dry ingredients in a large electric mixer bowl. With the mixer running at low speed, gradually add the liquid mixture and oil. Beat the dough for three minutes at medium speed. Scrape the dough from the beaters and the sides of the bowl into the bottom of the bowl. It will be very sticky. Oil the top of the dough and the sides of the bowl, and cover the bowl with a towel. Put the bowl in a warm (85°F to 90°F) place* and let the dough rise for 1 to 1½ hours. Beat the dough again for three minutes at medium speed.

Oil and flour an 8 by 4 inch loaf pan. Put the dough in the pan and allow it to rise in a warm place for about 20 to 35* minutes, or until it barely doubles. Preheat the oven to 375°F. Bake the loaf for about 50 to 65 minutes, loosely covering it with foil after the first 30 to 45 minutes if it is getting excessively brown. Remove the loaf from the pan and cool it completely on a cooling rack. Makes one loaf.

*Notes: On eggs: If you are allergic to eggs, use ¾ cup warm water in their place. If you do not take the eggs out of the refrigerator early enough for them to come to room temperature before you are ready to bake, put them in a bowl of warm water for 5 or 10 minutes before cracking them to use in this recipe.

On guar or xanthum gum: When making the dough for this bread in a bread machine, mix together the guar or xanthum gum and flour before adding them to the machine. If you just add the ingredients to the machine in the order listed, during the warm-up time before mixing begins, the water and gum can form lumps that routine mixing may not completely eliminate.

On the final rise before baking: If you are making this bread using a programmable bread machine, set the last rise to 25 minutes.

On a warm rising place: To use your oven as a cozy place for bread to rise, see the third paragraph on page 179.

Spelt Bread

When made with white spelt, this bread is so normal in taste and texture that guests may be surprised that they are not eating wheat. It can be made on the basic bread cycle of any bread machine. Always use Purity Foods™ flour to make spelt yeast bread. Refer to page 54 to read why.

> 1 cup water
> ¼ cup apple juice concentrate, thawed
> 1½ tablespoons oil
> 1 teaspoon salt
> About 3¼ to 3¾ cups whole spelt flour or 4½ to 5¼ cups white spelt
>   flour*
> 2¼ teaspoons (1 package) active dry yeast

To make this recipe with a bread machine, add the ingredients to the pan in the order listed using the smaller amount of the flour. Chose the basic cycle and a loaf size of 1½ pounds for whole spelt bread or 2 pounds for white spelt bread. Start the machine. After a few minutes of mixing, look in the machine. If the dough is very soft, begin adding more flour about 2 tablespoons at a time until it reaches a consistency that is not sticky. After about 10 minutes of mixing, re-check the consistency of the dough and add flour if needed. It should not be too soft or sticky and be starting to become elastic. Re-check the dough near the end of the kneading time, such as when the "add raisins" timer sounds, because it can soften with kneading and may need more flour. Then allow the rest of the cycle to run.

To make this recipe with a mixer, put one-half to two-thirds of the flour, the yeast, and the salt in the mixer bowl. Mix on low speed for about 30 seconds. Warm the liquid ingredients to 115 to 120°F. With the mixer running on low speed, add the liquids to the dry ingredients in a slow stream. Continue mixing until the dry and liquid ingredients are thoroughly mixed. If your mixer is not a heavy-duty mixer, at this point beat the dough for 5 to 10 minutes. You will be able to tell that the gluten is developing because the dough will begin to climb up the beaters. Then knead the rest of the flour in by hand, kneading for about 10 minutes, or until the dough is very smooth and elastic.

If your mixer is a heavy-duty mixer, after the liquids are thoroughly mixed in, with the mixer still running, begin adding the rest of the flour around the edges of the bowl ½ cup at a time, mixing well after each addition before adding more flour, until the dough forms a ball and cleans the sides of the bowl. Knead the dough on the speed directed in your mixer manual for 5 to 10 minutes or until the dough is very elastic and smooth. If it softens during kneading, add more flour. Turn the dough out onto a floured board and knead it briefly to check the consistency of the dough, kneading in a little more flour if necessary.

Put the dough into an oiled bowl and turn it once so that the top of the ball is also oiled. Cover it with a towel and let it rise in a warm (85°F to 90°F) place* until it has doubled in volume, about 45 minutes to 1 hour.

While the dough is rising, prepare your baking pan. Spelt flour is different than any other flour in that it can be very difficult to get the bread out of the pan. (This may be because spelt is more soluble than other flours. See page 219 for more about this). Rub the inside of an 8-inch by 4-inch or 9-inch by 5-inch loaf pan with oil. Cut a piece of parchment or waxed paper the length of the pan and put it in the pan so the bottom and sides are covered with the paper. Oil the paper also.

When the dough has doubled in volume, punch it down and shape it into a loaf. Put the loaf into the prepared loaf pan. Allow it to rise until double again. Bake bread at 375°F for 45 minutes to an hour or until it is nicely browned. Check it midway through the baking time, and if it is already getting brown, cover it with a piece of foil to prevent over-browning. At the end of the baking time, remove the loaf from the pan. You may need to run a knife along the ends of the pan which are not lined with paper to loosen the loaf. If it is done, it should sound hollow when tapped on the bottom. Cool it completely on a cooling rack before slicing it. If you can't wait to eat it, slice it carefully with a serrated knife. Makes one loaf.

*Notes: Even if you use Purity Foods™ flour, spelt flour is variable from batch to batch on how much flour it takes to make dough of the right consistency. Most bread machine recipes do not require much adjustment, and gluten-free recipes should be made "as written" the first time, because their dough may be the consistency of a stiff batter. However, in this recipe, you may have to check the dough several times throughout the kneading time and add more flour.

On a warm rising place: To use your oven as a cozy place for bread to rise, see the third paragraph on page 179.

Quick and Easy All-Fruit Desserts

Sometimes we want a sweet treat and we want it now! You can have it using the recipes in this chapter. Keep a can of pineapple in your freezer at all times, and you will be able to have pineapple sorbet within a few minutes whenever the craving for something sweet hits. The recipes in this chapter are made from fruit, so they are tops for nutrition as well as for speed and ease.

Banana Sorbet

Gluten-Free

Do you ever find yourself with too many bananas ripening at one time? You hate to let them go to waste but don't have time to bake banana bread. Peel them, break them into chunks, and put them in plastic bags to store in the freezer. (I like to put each banana in a small sandwich bag and store the small bags in a larger Ziploc™ bag). Then when you want a quick dessert, you will have frozen bananas on hand to make this delicious sugar-free sorbet. Top with chocolate sauce, below, for a real treat!

> 2 large bananas
> 2 to 3 tablespoons agave, Fruit Sweet™ or honey, to taste (optional)

Cut the bananas into chunks, put the chunks into a plastic bag and freeze them for several hours or overnight, or you may store them in the freezer for an extended period of time. When you are ready to have the sorbet, remove them from the freezer and let them stand at room temperature for 10 minutes. Blend with a hand blender until smooth or puree them with a food processor or standard blender. Taste the sorbet and blend in the sweetener if desired. Serve immediately for a smooth, creamy dessert. Freeze any leftovers. Remove the leftovers from the freezer about 20 minutes before serving. Makes 2 to 4 servings.

Chocolate Sauce: Melt two 1-ounce squares of unsweetened baking chocolate in a double boiler over simmering water or in your microwave oven. To melt chocolate in the microwave, place it in a glass bowl and microwave it, breaking-ing it up and stirring it at 30-second intervals, until it is mostly melted with just a few solid parts remaining. Remove it from the microwave and stir it to melt the remaining solid chocolate. Add ½ cup of agave to the chocolate and blend with a hand blender or blender. Serve immediately or refrigerate. This sauce will become quite thick when refrigerated; microwave it for a few seconds and stir it to liquefy it for serving.

Pineapple Sorbet

Gluten-Free

You can't get much easier than a recipe that contains only one ingredient!

1 20-ounce can of pineapple chunks or tidbits packed in their own juice

Put the can of pineapple in the freezer and let it freeze for several hours or overnight, or you may store it in the freezer for an extended period of time and have it ready for sorbet whenever the mood strikes. When you are ready to have sorbet, remove the can of pineapple from the freezer and run hot water over it or let it stand at room temperature for 10 to 20 minutes. Open the can on both ends and push the pineapple out. Put about half of the can into the cup that came with your hand blender and blend it with the hand blender until smooth. Do the same with the other half-can of pineapple. (If you use a food processor or standard blender, use it to easily puree the whole can at one time). Serve immediately for a smooth, creamy dessert. Freeze any leftovers. Remove the leftovers from the freezer about 20 minutes before serving. Makes 3 to 6 servings.

Cherry or Berry-Banana Sorbet

Gluten-Free

This is simple to make from frozen berries without needing to freeze bananas in advance. However, if you have frozen bananas you want to use, let them thaw for about 10 minutes and then you can use them in this recipe.

2 ripe bananas
2 tablespoons agave, honey or Fruit Sweet™ (optional)
4 to 6 cups frozen dark (Bing) cherries, strawberries, blueberries, or
    raspberries

Puree the bananas and optional sweetener in a food processor or blender or blend with a hand blender until smooth. Gradually add the cherries or berries, processing after each addition, until the sorbet reaches the desired consistency. Serve immediately. Freeze any leftovers. Remove the leftovers from the freezer about 20 minutes before serving. Makes about 4 cups of sorbet, or 6 to 8 servings.

Baked Apples or Pears

Gluten-Free

This homey dessert is wonderful as part of an oven meal.

    4 large baking apples* or pears
    ½ cup thawed apple juice concentrate, apple juice, pear juice, or water
        OR ¼ cup agave, Fruit Sweet™ or honey plus ¼ cup water
    ½ teaspoon cinnamon (optional)
    ¼ cup raisins (optional)

Core the apples or pears and put them in a 2½ quart glass casserole dish with a lid. Pour in the juice, sweetener, and/or water and sprinkle the cinnamon down the centers of the fruit. Stuff the fruit with raisins, if desired. Bake at 350°F for 40 to 50 minutes for the apples or 1 to 1½ hours for the pears or until the fruit is tender when pierced with a fork. Makes 4 servings.

*Note on baking apples: Some varieties of apples hold their shape well when they are baked, such as Rome, Pink Lady, and Granny Smith. If you're planning to make this dessert for guests and will be buying the apples especially for baking, chose a baking apple. However, if you have old apples in your refrigerator that you want to use up, any kind will be fine to use in this recipe.

Quick and Easy Fruit Tapioca

Gluten-Free

This dessert is easy to make using canned fruit and is great as part of an oven meal.

    1 16 to 20-ounce can of fruit, such as juice-packed sliced peaches, pears
        or pineapple chunks, not drained, OR water-packed pie cherries,
        drained
    ¼ cup quick-cooking (minute) tapioca
    1 cup water or fruit juice for the peaches, pears, or pineapple, or 1 cup
        apple juice concentrate plus ½ cup water for the cherries

Combine all of the ingredients in a 1½-quart casserole dish. Bake at 350°F for 40 to 60 minutes or until the tapioca is clear. Makes 4 servings.

Fruit Tapioca Pudding

Gluten-Free

Although this recipe is not quite a speedy and the previous recipe, if you have fresh fruit you need to use up, this is the one for you. To use up an abundance of ripening fruit, double or triple the recipe and freeze the leftovers.

1½ to 2 pounds of apples, peaches, or nectarines
½ cup apple juice concentrate, thawed
1½ tablespoons quick-cooking (minute) tapioca
¾ teaspoon cinnamon with the apples or ⅛ teaspoon nutmeg with
     the peaches or nectarines

Peel, core, and slice the fruit to produce about 9 or 10 cups of slices.

To cook this dessert on the stove top, combine ¼ cup of the apple juice concentrate, the fruit, and the spice in a large saucepan. Bring them to a boil over medium heat, reduce the heat, and simmer until the fruit is tender, about 15 to 25 minutes Near the end of the cooking time, combine the tapioca with the remaining ¼ cup apple juice concentrate and allow it to stand for at least 5 minutes. Stir the tapioca mixture into the fruit when it is tender. Return the pan to a boil, and simmer for an additional 5 minutes. Let stand for at least 20 minutes before serving.

To cook this dessert in the oven as part of an oven meal, combine the peeled and sliced fruit, tapioca, juice and spice in a 1½-quart casserole dish. Bake at 350°F for 40 to 60 minutes, or until the tapioca is clear. Makes 4 servings.

Special Desserts and Cookies

Let's face it – sweet treats are enjoyable, and a celiac or food allergy diet usually should not mean that we have to go through life without them. Desserts can be made from inexpensive healthy ingredients, and some can be made without spending much time. In this chapter you will find recipes for sweet treats that will fit into your food allergy or gluten-free diet. Many of them are so quick and easy to make that you will be enjoying them in less time than it takes to go out and shop for a store-bought treat instead. All of them will save you money over their commercially-made counterparts and taste better because they are freshly made.

Aside from the sugar-free whipped cream recipe, the desserts and cookies in this chapter do not require an electric mixer; you can mix them with a spoon. The procedure for making them is the same as for quick breads. See pages 62 and 63 for instructions on how to mix these cookie and cake recipes.

Some of the recipes in this chapter require a blender of some kind. See pages 42 to 43 for information about hand blenders. If you have a standard blender or food processor, you can use it instead.

If your allergies are so extensive that you cannot find desserts you can eat in this chapter or if you need stevia-sweetened treats because of candidiasis, see *The Ultimate Food Allergy Cookbook and Survival Guide* as described on the last pages of this book.

Cookies

Chocolate Brownies

Gluten-Free

These chewy brownies have been favorites of everyone who tasted them. You'll have a hard time believing that they are gluten and grain-free.

2 1-ounce squares of unsweetened chocolate
⅜ cup oil
1 cup white cane or beet sugar or fine maple sugar
2 large eggs
½ teaspoon salt
¾ cup buckwheat flour
½ teaspoon GF baking powder

Preheat your oven to 350°F. Oil an 8-inch square metal baking pan. Line the bottom and two opposite sides of the pan with an 8-inch wide strip of parchment or waxed paper. Also oil the paper. Melt the chocolate in a double boiler over boiling water or carefully microwave it in a glass bowl, stirring often, until it is just melted. Stir the oil into the melted chocolate thoroughly. Add the sugar, eggs, and salt and stir thoroughly. In a separate bowl, stir together the flour and baking powder. Add the dry ingredients to the chocolate mixture and stir until just mixed. Spread the batter in the prepared pan. Bake for 30 minutes or until the top has a dull crust and a toothpick inserted into the brownies comes out with just a few moist crumbs on it. Cool in the pan. Then cut into squares. Makes 16 brownies.

Carob Brownies

Gluten-Free

These gluten and grain-free fruit-sweetened brownies are a delicious and satisfying treat for those who must avoid chocolate.

1 cup amaranth flour
¼ cup arrowroot
⅓ cup carob powder
½ teaspoon baking soda
¾ cup apple juice concentrate, thawed
¼ cup oil

Preheat your oven to 350°F. Oil and flour a 9 inch by 5 inch metal loaf pan. If your carob powder contains lumps, press it through a strainer with the back of a spoon to remove the lumps before measuring it. Combine the amaranth flour, arrowroot, carob powder, and baking soda in a bowl. In another bowl or measuring cup, stir together the apple juice concentrate and oil. Stir the liquid ingredients into the dry ingredients until just mixed and immediately put the batter into the prepared pan. Bake for 20 minutes. The batter will puff up during baking and then collapse either near the end of the baking time or after you remove the brownies from the oven. Do not overbake. The toothpick test on page 63 does not apply to these brownies; if you test them with a toothpick, the toothpick will come out with wet dough on it. These brownies have a moist, chewy texture. At the end of the baking time, remove the pan from the oven and cool the brownies completely before cutting. Makes 8 to 10 brownies.

Choose Your Chip Cookies

Gluten-Free IF
made with a GF grain

This recipe can be made with your choice of three grains and a variety of additions including chocolate chips such as Enjoy Life™ chips which are gluten, dairy, and soy-free. For more varieties of chip cookies (millet, sorghum, teff, buckwheat, rye, barley, whole spelt, kamut, etc.) see the next two recipes and The Ultimate Food Allergy Cookbook and Survival Guide *described on the last pages of this book.*

Amaranth (GF):

2¼ cups amaranth flour

¾ cup arrowroot

1 teaspoon baking soda

¼ teaspoon unbuffered vitamin C powder

¼ teaspoon salt

1¼ cup apple juice concentrate, thawed

¼ cup oil

¾ cup chocolate or carob chips, raisins or other chopped dried fruit, or chopped nuts (optional)

Quinoa (GF):

2 cups quinoa flour

⅔ cup tapioca starch

2½ teaspoons GF baking powder OR 1 teaspoons baking soda plus ¼ teaspoon unbuffered vitamin C powder

⅞ cup agave or Fruit Sweet™

⅓ cup oil

1 cup chocolate or carob chips, raisins or other chopped dried fruit, or chopped nuts (optional)

White Spelt:

3½ cups white spelt flour

1 teaspoon baking powder plus ½ teaspoon baking soda OR 1 teaspoon baking soda plus ¼ teaspoon unbuffered vitamin C powder

½ teaspoon salt

1 cup agave, Fruit Sweet™ or honey

1 cup oil

2 teaspoons vanilla extract (optional)

1 cup chocolate or carob chips, raisins or other chopped dried fruit, or chopped nuts (optional)

Preheat your oven to 350°F for the quinoa cookies or 375°F for the other cookies. If you are using the agave, line your baking sheets with parchment paper. In a large bowl stir together the flour(s), baking soda, vitamin C, and/or baking powder and salt. In a separate bowl or measuring cup thoroughly combine the sweetener, oil, and optional vanilla extract. Stir the liquid ingredients into the dry ingredients until they are just mixed. Fold in the chocolate or carob chips or other additions. Drop the batter by heaping teaspoonfuls 2 to 3 inches apart on the baking sheets. Bake the cookies for 9 to 15 minutes or until they are golden brown. Remove them from the baking sheets with a spatula and put them on paper towels to cool. Makes 3 to 4 dozen cookies.

Millet or Teff Apple Cookies

Gluten-Free

The teff-cinnamon variety of these cookies is delicious! And although they are fragile, the millet cookies are especially good when made with carob or chocolate chips.

> 2 cups millet or teff flour
> ½ teaspoon baking soda
> 1 teaspoon cinnamon (optional – omit with the carob or chocolate chips)
> ½ cup unsweetened applesauce
> 2 extra-large eggs (about ½ cup in volume), lightly beaten
> ½ cup agave or Fruit Sweet™
> ⅓ cup oil
> ¾ cup chocolate or carob chips, raisins or other chopped dried fruit, or chopped nuts (optional)

Preheat your oven to 350°F. If you are using the agave, line your baking sheets with parchment paper. Combine the flour, baking soda, and cinnamon in a large bowl. Lightly beat the eggs with a fork and combine them with the applesauce, sweetener, and oil. Mix the liquids together thoroughly and then stir them into the flour mixture until they are just mixed in. Quickly fold in the nuts or carob chips. Drop the batter by heaping teaspoonfuls onto an ungreased baking sheet. Bake for 15 to 20 minutes, or until the cookies begin to brown. Remove them from the baking sheet with a spatula and cool them on paper towels. Makes about 3½ dozen cookies.

No egg, all apple variation: Omit the eggs and use 1 cup apple juice concentrate, thawed, instead of the eggs and agave or Fruit Sweet™.

Gingersnaps

3 cups barley flour
1 teaspoon baking soda
¼ teaspoon unbuffered vitamin C powder
¼ teaspoon salt
½ teaspoon ginger (omit with the chocolate or carob chips)
1 cup light molasses or agave (Agave is best with the chocolate or carob chips).
½ cup oil
1 cup chocolate or carob chips, raisins or other chopped dried fruit, or chopped nuts (optional)

Preheat your oven to 350°F. If you are using the agave, line your baking sheets with parchment paper. Combine the flour, baking soda, salt, and ginger in a large bowl. Mix the sweetener and oil together thoroughly and then stir them into the flour mixture until they are just mixed in. Quickly fold in the chocolate chips or other additions. Drop the batter by heaping teaspoonfuls onto the baking sheets. Flatten the cookies to about ¼ inch thickness with your fingers if you prefer them thin. Bake for 10 to15 minutes, or until the cookies begin to brown. Remove them from the baking sheet with a spatula and cool them on paper towels. Makes about 3 dozen cookies.

Quinoa Almond Cookies

Gluten-Free

This cookie has several different personalities depending on what you use for the sweetener. Try all the varieties – each is delicious in its own unique way.

1½ cups quinoa flour
2¼ teaspoons GF baking powder OR ¾ teaspoon baking soda plus ¼ teaspoon unbuffered vitamin C powder
½ cup almond meal/flour (See "Sources," page 213).
¼ cup sliced almonds (optional)
½ cup oil
½ teaspoon almond flavoring
½ cup agave or honey (for crisp cookies) OR ½ cup agave or honey plus ½ cup water (for soft cookies) OR 1 cup apple juice concentrate, thawed (for fruit-sweetened soft cookies)

Preheat your oven to 375°. If you are using the agave, line your baking sheets with parchment paper. Combine the flour, baking powder or baking soda plus vitamin C, almond meal, and almonds in a large bowl. Thoroughly mix the oil with the sweetener, sweetener plus water, or juice in a measuring cup or small bowl. Immediately pour the liquids into the dry ingredients. Stir the dough until it is just mixed. Drop it by teaspoonfuls onto an ungreased baking sheet. For the crisp cookies, flatten the cookies with your fingers held together. Bake the cookies at 375°F for 7 to 10 minutes. Remove them from the baking sheet with a spatula and cool them on paper towels. Makes about 2 dozen crisp or 3 dozen soft cookies.

Very crisp and flaky variation: Make the crisp cookie variation of this recipe using ½ cup agave or honey (without the water) for the sweetener and also decrease the flour to 1 cup. You will not need to flatten the cookies with your fingers or a glass because the batter will be much thinner and will spread readily. Place the cookies at least 3 to 4 inches apart on the baking sheet. Bake as above.

Tropical Delights

1 cup pineapple canned in its own juice with the juice (crushed, chunks, or tidbits work well)
2 cups rye flour or 2⅛ cups white spelt flour
½ teaspoon baking soda
¼ teaspoon salt
1 cup unsweetened shredded coconut
¾ cup pineapple juice concentrate, thawed
½ cup oil

Preheat your oven to 375°F. Lightly oil two to three baking sheets. Put the pineapple in a 2-cup measuring cup and puree it with a hand blender, or puree it with a food processor or standard blender. Add the pineapple juice concentrate and oil and puree again briefly. In a large bowl, stir together the flour, baking soda, salt, and coconut. Stir the liquid ingredients into the dry ingredients until they are just mixed. Drop the batter by heaping teaspoonfuls 2 to 3 inches apart on the prepared baking sheets. Bake the cookies for 15 to 19 minutes or until they are golden brown on the bottom and just beginning to brown on the top. Remove them from the baking sheets and put them on paper towels to cool. Makes about 3 dozen cookies.

Shortbread

Gluten-Free IF
made with a GF grain

These cookies are easy to make with a wide variety of flours which adds variety to a celiac diet or makes shortbread fit any day of an allergy rotation diet. For several more varieties made with other flours, see The Ultimate Food Allergy Cookbook and Survival Guide *as described on the last pages of this book.*

Amaranth (GF):

1¼ cups amaranth flour
1 cup arrowroot
½ teaspoon baking soda
⅜ cup oil
½ cup pineapple juice concentrate, thawed

Quinoa (GF):

1¼ cups quinoa flour
1 cup tapioca starch
½ teaspoon baking soda
⅜ cup oil
½ cup apple juice concentrate, thawed

Date-Oat*:

2¼ cups oat flour
½ cup date sugar, pressed through a strainer to remove any lumps
½ teaspoon baking soda
⅛ teaspoon unbuffered vitamin C powder
⅜ cup oil
½ cup water

Pineapple-Oat*:

2½ cups oat flour
½ teaspoon baking soda
⅜ cup oil
½ cup pineapple juice concentrate, thawed

Teff (GF):

2 cups teff flour

1½ teaspoons GF baking powder OR ½ teaspoon baking soda plus ⅛
   teaspoon vitamin C powder

½ cup oil

¼ cup Fruit Sweet™ or agave

1 large egg plus enough water to bring its volume up to ¼ cup OR ¼
   cup water

Barley:

2 cups barley flour

½ teaspoon baking soda

⅜ cup oil

½ cup apple juice concentrate, thawed

Whole Spelt:

1½ cups whole spelt flour

1 cup arrowroot or tapioca flour

½ teaspoon baking soda

⅜ cup oil

½ cup apple juice concentrate, thawed

White Spelt:

1½ cups white spelt flour

1 cup cornstarch, tapioca starch, or arrowroot

½ teaspoon baking soda

¼ teaspoon salt

½ cup oil

⅜ cup Fruit Sweet™, agave, or slightly warmed honey

Choose one set of ingredients above. Preheat your oven to 350°F. If you are using the agave or making white spelt shortbread, line your baking sheet with parchment paper. Combine the flour(s), baking powder, baking soda, and/or vitamin C powder, and date sugar (if you are using it) in a large bowl. Stir together the oil and sweetener or water and add them to the dry ingredients, mixing with a spoon and your hands until the dough sticks together. If necessary, add another 1 to 2 tablespoons of water or juice to help it stick together. Roll the dough out to ¼ inch thickness on a baking sheet and cut it into 1-inch by 2 to 3-inch rectangular bars. Bake until the cookies begin to brown. This will take about 15 to 20 minutes for the amaranth, quinoa, teff, oat, and spelt varieties and 20 to 25 minutes for the barley cookies. Take the baking sheet from the oven and re-cut the shortbread on the lines where it was previously cut. Remove the shortbread from the baking sheet with a spatula and put it on paper towels to cool. Makes 2½ to 3 dozen bars.

*Note: Some doctors allow their celiac patients to eat oats and others do not. Ask your doctor before eating the oat varieties of shortbread.

Desserts

Easy Fruit Crumble

Ask your doctor.

This recipe is as easy to make as it is delicious. Although millet flakes are currently unavailable in the United States, perhaps the rising number of people on gluten-free diets will convince an entrepreneur or company to begin importing them again. Or if you have a British friend, ask him or her to send you some. If you can eat oats, this dessert is also delicious made with oatmeal.

> 4 cups fresh blueberries or peeled and sliced apples or peaches
>   OR 4 cups drained water-packed canned peaches or apples
>   OR 1 pound frozen blueberries
> ¾ to 1 cup date sugar, divided
> ¼ cup arrowroot or tapioca starch
> 2 to 6 tablespoons water, divided
> 1 cup millet flakes or oatmeal, uncooked
> 1 teaspoon cinnamon
> ¼ cup oil

Preheat your oven to 325°F. Taste the fruit you are going to use. If it is sweet, use ¼ cup date sugar with the fruit. If it is tart, use ½ cup date sugar with the fruit. Combine the ¼ or ½ cup date sugar and the arrowroot or tapioca starch in an 8 inch square baking dish. Stir the fruit into the date sugar mixture. If you are using fresh fruit, sprinkle 4 tablespoons water over the blueberries or apples. Sprinkle 2 tablespoons water over fresh peaches, canned apples, or frozen blueberries. No water is needed with canned peaches.

In a small bowl, combine the cereal, remaining ½ cup date sugar, and cinnamon. Stir in the oil until the mixture is crumbly. Stir in 2 tablespoons of water.

Sprinkle the mixture on top of the fruit. Bake for 30 to 40 minutes or until the topping browns and the fruit is tender when pierced with a fork. Makes 6 to 8 servings.

*Note: Some doctors allow their celiac patients to eat oats and others do not. Ask your doctor before eating the oat variety of this dessert. If you use millet flakes to make this dessert, it is gluten-free.

No-Grain Easy Fruit Crumble

Gluten-Free

This is my favorite dessert with its pairing of sumptuous fruit and a crunchy topping.

> 4 cups fresh blueberries or peeled and sliced apples or peaches
> OR 4 cups drained water-packed canned peaches or apples
> OR 1 pound frozen blueberries
> ¼ cup arrowroot or tapioca starch
> ½ to ¾ cup date sugar, divided
> Up to 4 tablespoons water
> ¼ cup almond meal/flour or pecan meal/flour (See "Sources," page 213).
> ⅔ cup unsweetened coconut
> ⅓ cup chopped or sliced almonds or chopped pecans
> Cinnamon – 1¼ teaspoon with the apples, ¼ teaspoon with the other fruit
> ¼ cup oil

Preheat your oven to 375°F. Combine the fruit, arrowroot or tapioca starch, 1 teaspoon cinnamon (with the apples only), and ¼ to ½ cup of date sugar (depending on how sweet the fruit is) in a deep 8 or 9 inch square baking dish or 2 to 3-quart casserole dish. Add just enough water to barely moisten the starch and date sugar. The starch-liquid mixture should be like a thick paste. How much water you will need to add will depend on how juicy your fruit is; with canned peaches you will not need to add any water.

In a bowl, stir together the remaining ¼ cup date sugar, nut meal, coconut, nuts, and ¼ teaspoon cinnamon. Pour the oil over the mixture and stir until it is evenly distributed. Sprinkle the nut mixture over the fruit in the baking dish. Bake for 10 minutes. Then cover it with foil to prevent excessive browning. Bake for another 35 to 45 minutes or until the filling is bubbly throughout. Makes about 6 servings.

Easy Apple Crisp

Ask your doctor.

You can make this guest-worthy dessert quickly with water-packed canned sliced apples, such as Mussleman's™ brand. For variety, use fresh seasonal fruits such as peaches or blueberries instead.

Filling ingredients:

> 2 20-ounce cans of sliced apples canned in water, drained
> 1 tablespoon plus 1 teaspoon cornstarch, arrowroot, or tapioca starch
> 1½ teaspoons cinnamon
> ⅓ cup apple juice concentrate, thawed

Topping ingredients:

> ¾ cup oatmeal, quick cooking or regular (not instant)
> ¾ cup white spelt or rice flour
> ½ teaspoon baking soda
> ¼ cup oil
> ¼ cup agave or Fruit Sweet™ OR 3 tablespoons honey plus 1 tablespoon water
> 1 teaspoon vanilla extract

Drain the canned apples. Put the slices in a 2½ to 3-quart glass casserole dish. Add the starch and cinnamon and toss with the apple slices to coat the slices thoroughly. Drizzle the apple juice concentrate over the apple slices.

Preheat your oven to 350°F. In a mixing bowl, stir together the oatmeal, flour, and baking soda. If you are using the honey, warm it slightly and mix it well with the water. In a cup, combine the sweetener, oil, and vanilla. Stir them into the dry ingredients until just mixed. Drop and spread the topping over the apples in the casserole dish. Bake the dish for 25 to 40 minutes or until the apples are tender and bubbling and the topping is browned. Check the apple crisp after 30 minutes; if the topping is already getting quite brown but the fruit is not done, cover it with foil for the rest of the baking time. Makes 6 to 8 servings.

Fresh Peach Crisp Variation: Substitute 10 to 12 peaches weighing about 3 pounds, peeled, cored, and sliced, for the canned apples and increase the amount of apple juice concentrate you use in the filling to ½ cup.

Blueberry Crisp Variation: Substitute 2 pounds of fresh or frozen blueberries for the canned apples and omit the cinnamon.

Fresh Apple Crisp Variation: Substitute 8 large apples weighing about 3 pounds for the canned apples. Peel, core and slice the apples and put them in a saucepan with 1½ cups of water. Cover the pan and bring the apple slices to a boil. Reduce the heat to medium, and simmer them for 5 to 10 minutes or until they just begin to soften. Drain the apple slices and use them in the recipe above.

Note: If your doctor allows oats on a celiac diet, you should be able to have this dessert if made with the rice flour. Ask your doctor before eating this dessert.

Quick-Mix No-Roll Pie Crust

Gluten-Free IF made with a GF grain

Are the holidays coming? No problem! You can easily make a special diet pie. Here are three varieties of a quick-to-make pie crust to go with the fillings on the next three pages The amaranth crust has a delicious nutty taste. If you are allergic to wheat rather than gluten-intolerant, the spelt crust is near normal and will be enjoyed by guests. The rice crust is bland-tasting, but is included for celiacs who are not into amaranth.

Amaranth (GF):

> 1½ cups amaranth flour
> ¾ cup arrowroot
> ½ teaspoon salt
> ½ teaspoon GF baking powder
> ⅝ cup oil
> ¼ cup cold water

Rice (GF):

> 3 cups rice flour
> ½ teaspoon salt
> ½ teaspoon GF baking powder
> ¼ teaspoon cinnamon (optional)
> ⅔ cup oil
> ⅓ cup cold water or apple juice

White Spelt:

> 2¾ cups white spelt flour
> ½ teaspoon salt
> ½ teaspoon baking powder
> ½ cup oil
> ¼ cup cold water

Chose one set of ingredients on the previous page. In a large bowl, stir together the flour(s), salt, baking powder, and optional cinnamon. Measure the water or juice and oil into the same measuring cup and stir them together thoroughly. Before they have a chance to separate, pour them into the bowl with the flour. Stir the ingredients together quickly; if the flour does not all incorporate into the dough readily, cut the mixture with the side of the spoon to help it come into a crumbly mixture. Do not stir or cut the dough for very long; you should not over-work the dough.

For two one-crust pies, press half of the dough on to the bottom and sides of each of two pie plates. Preheat your oven to 400°F. Bake for 10 to 15 minutes or until the pie crust is lightly browned.

For a two-crust pie, press half of the dough on to the bottom and sides of pie plate, add the filling, and crumble the other half of the dough over the filling. Bake as directed in the filling recipe.

Makes two single pie crusts or enough crust for a two-crust pie.

Blueberry Pie

Gluten-Free IF made with a GF crust

This pie is quick, easy, and convenient to make using frozen blueberries.

> 1½ pounds fresh or frozen unsweetened blueberries
> 1 cup of apple juice concentrate, thawed
> 3 tablespoons cornstarch, arrowroot, or tapioca starch OR 5 tablespoons quick cooking (minute) tapioca
> 1 baked single pie crust OR 1 batch of pastry for a two-crust pie, recipe on page 167

Combine the apple juice concentrate and thickener in a saucepan. If you are using the minute tapioca, let it stand for five minutes before you begin cooking it. Add the blueberries to the pan and stir. Heat the fruit mixture over low to medium heat, stirring frequently, until it comes to a boil and thickens.

For a one-crust pie, cool the filling for ten minutes before putting it into the baked and cooled crust. Refrigerate the pie.

For a two-crust pie, while the fruit is cooking, preheat your oven to 400°F. Put the filling into the unbaked bottom pie crust. Cover the filling with the top crust. Bake the pie at 400°F for 10 minutes; then reduce the heat to 350°F and continue to bake it for another 40 to 50 minutes or until the top and bottom crusts are golden brown. Makes 6 to 8 servings.

Apple Pie

Gluten-Free IF
made with a GF crust

You will never miss the sugar in this all time favorite pie. For other fruit-sweetened pie fillings (peach, cherry, grape, coconut, etc.) see The Ultimate Food Allergy Cookbook and Survival Guide *as described on the last pages of this book.*

> 6 to 7 apples, peeled, cored and sliced to make about 5 cups of slices or
> 1½ 20-ounce cans of water-packed apple slices such as Mussleman's™
> brand, drained
> ⅝ cup apple juice concentrate, thawed
> 1 teaspoon cinnamon
> An additional ¼ cup of apple juice concentrate, thawed
> 2 tablespoons cornstarch, arrowroot, or tapioca starch OR 3 tablespoons
> of quick cooking (minute) tapioca
> Pastry for a two crust pie, recipe on page 167

If you are using the canned apples, thoroughly drain the water from the cans. Combine the apple slices, ⅝ cup apple juice concentrate, and cinnamon in a saucepan. Bring them to a boil and reduce the heat to a simmer. For fresh apples, simmer for about 15 to 20 minutes. If you are using canned apples, simmer for a minute or two to heat them. While they are cooking, in a separate cup stir together the additional ¼ cup apple juice concentrate with the starch or tapioca. If you are using minute tapioca, let it stand for 5 minutes in the juice. Stir the starch mixture into the saucepan at the end of the simmering time for the apples. Continue to cook on medium heat until the fruit mixture returns to a boil and thickens.

While the fruit is cooking, preheat your oven to 400°F. Put the filling into the unbaked bottom pie crust. Cover the filling with the top crust. Bake the pie at 400°F for 10 minutes; then reduce the heat to 350°F and continue to bake it for another 40 to 50 minutes or until the top and bottom crusts are golden brown. Makes 6 to 8 servings.

Sugar-Free Whipped Cream

Gluten-Free

> 1 cup heavy or whipping cream
> 2 to 4 teaspoons of Fruit Sweet™, agave, or honey, to taste.

Get out the electric mixer; this is the rare time when you really need to use it. Pour the whipping cream into the narrow bowl and beat it at the whipped cream setting. Whip it until soft peaks form. Add sweetener to your taste and continue to whip it until the peaks become firm. Serve immediately. Makes 8 to 12 servings.

No Bake Pumpkin Pie

Gluten-Free IF
made with a GF crust

Here is an easy, allergen-free pie for Thanksgiving. If you have no Candida or other intestinal dysbiosis problems and want a lighter colored pie, use brown or white sugar in place of the date sugar.

    1 16-ounce can of plain pumpkin
    1 cup water
    1 envelope unflavored gelatin
    1 cup date sugar
    1 teaspoon cinnamon
    1 teaspoon nutmeg
    ¼ teaspoon cloves
    ¼ teaspoon allspice
    ¼ teaspoon ginger
    1 baked single-crust pie shell, recipe on page 167
    Sugar-free whipped cream, recipe on page 169 (optional)

Prepare and bake the pie shell. Put the water in a saucepan and sprinkle the gelatin over the surface of the water. Heat the water over medium heat, stirring occasionally, until it comes to a boil and the gelatin dissolves. Stir in the rest of the ingredients. Put the pumpkin mixture into the pie shell and refrigerate it for several hours until it is thoroughly chilled. Serve with whipped cream if desired and if you tolerate dairy products. Makes 6 to 8 servings.

Gingerbread

Gluten-Free IF
made with a GF grain

This is wonderful served from the baking pan with whipped cream. See the sugar-free whipped cream recipe on page 169.

Amaranth (GF):

    1½ cups amaranth flour
    ½ cup arrowroot
    1 teaspoon baking soda
    ¼ teaspoon unbuffered vitamin C powder
    ¾ teaspoon ginger
    1 teaspoon cinnamon

¾ cup molasses
¼ cup water
¼ cup oil

Quinoa (GF):

1¼ cups quinoa flour
½ cup tapioca starch
2½ teaspoons GF baking powder OR 1 teaspoon baking soda plus ¼
    teaspoon unbuffered vitamin C powder
¾ teaspoon ginger
1 teaspoon cinnamon
¾ cup molasses
¼ cup water
¼ cup oil

Spelt:

2 cups whole spelt flour
1 teaspoon baking soda
¼ teaspoon unbuffered vitamin C powder
¾ teaspoon ginger
1 teaspoon cinnamon
¾ cup molasses
¼ cup water
¼ cup oil

Chose one set of ingredients above or on the previous page. Preheat your oven to 350°F. Oil and flour an 8 or 9 inch square cake pan. Combine the flour(s), baking powder or baking soda plus vitamin C, and spices in a large bowl. Mix the molasses with the water until the molasses is dissolved. Then add the oil and mix thoroughly. Stir the liquid ingredients into the dry ingredients until they are just combined. Put the batter into the prepared baking pan. Bake the cake for 30 to 35 minutes, or until a toothpick inserted in its center comes out dry. Makes one cake, or about 9 servings. If you can tolerate dairy products, serve this with whipped cream. (See the recipe on page 169).

Beverages, Snacks and Fun Foods

Most people find it easier to control spending on the groceries they buy to make meals than they do to limit spending on snacks, beverages, and fun foods. These foods are often not bought on planned trips to the grocery store. Instead, they may come from a coffee shop or convenience store in single-serving sized packages. They are often low in nutritional value. Therefore, if your food budget is tight, these foods are a good place to economize.

As in grocery shopping for meals, the way to save money on snacks and fun foods is to plan ahead. If you are on a food allergy or gluten-free diet, your diet may also necessitate planning ahead. Most of us on special diets take snacks and/or our lunch from home when we leave. I always travel with nuts in my car so if I'm gone longer than I expect, I do not get too hungry. Fresh or dried fruit also makes a convenient take-along snack.

Beverages purchased away from home also are usually low in nutritional value and can be high in price. Many people spend $2 to $4 or more for coffee every morning on the way to work. In a year's time, this habit can cost you $500 to $1000 as well as the time you spend waiting in line for your coffee. If finances are tight, save coffee shop coffee for a treat with a friend on special occasions and consider other options for your morning java.

There are many delicious coffees that you can brew at home and take with you in an insulated travel cup. If you have an automatic coffee maker, get it out, clean it by running some vinegar and water through it, and you will be ready to enjoy good coffee while saving money. If you do not own an automatic machine, excellent coffee can also be made quickly with an inexpensive French drip coffee system. Melitta offers such a system for $2.99. All you have to do is add coffee to a filter, set it over your cup or mug, and pour boiling water into the top of the system. In a few minutes, you have delicious inexpensive coffee. You can also purchase a system with a built-in gold mesh filter ($12.95, and not using paper filters saves money and makes for quick set-up) or a larger Melitta system with a travel mug ($8.99). See "Sources," page 212, for more about purchasing any of these systems.

If time is really tight in the morning, consider using high-quality instant coffee. Mount Hagen instant coffee is rich-tasting yet inexpensive. Taking a double-sized cup of Mount Hagen with you to work every morning will cost about $57 per year for the coffee plus the price of whatever creamers or sweeteners you like to add. Another advantage of using Mount Hagen instant coffee is that you can control the amount of caffeine by mixing part regular and part decaffeinated coffee crystals in your cup or mug. You also can avoid both artificial sweeteners and a blood sugar rush by using agave, a low-glycemic index natural sweetener, in your coffee.

Tea is rich in antioxidants and easy to make at home. I keep some large glass fruit juice bottles for making iced tea. Hang two to four tea bags from the edge of the bottle, add boiling water, and put the bottle in the refrigerator for a few hours or overnight. You can make a large bottle of iced tea this way for just a few pennies. If you are avoiding caffeine, many herbal teas make delicious iced tea, or you may use decaffeinated tea bags.

Soda pop is a favorite cold beverage but not a bargain nutritionally. Diet soda is water plus an assortment of chemicals, and in regular soda you get a massive infusion of sugar with the chemicals. As an alternative, a recipe for fruit juice soda is included in this chapter. You can save glass beverage bottles from carbonated water and reuse them to take homemade fruit juice soda along when you will be away from home. If time is more of an issue than money and you want an all-fruit carbonated beverage for outings away from home, try Knudsen™ fruit spritzers.

A favorite treat is going out for dinner or bringing home a take-out meal. The health implications of restaurant food are discussed on pages 11 to 12 and 21 to 24. For many on special diets, eating out is a carefully planned rare treat rather than a common occurrence. If your budget is too tight to eat out as often as you would like to, consider having fun by going on a picnic (see page 24) or making pizza at home. For the price of about six take-out pizzas, you can purchase an inexpensive Sunbeam 5891 bread machine and use it to make the spelt or rice pizza recipes in this chapter at home with minimal effort. You will recoup your investment in even a large programmable Zojirushi BBCC-X20 machine after you have made about fifteen pizzas, and this machine can make many types of allergy breads with its programmable cycles and will serve you faithfully for many years. Try making pizza by hand once or twice with the recipe found at the end of this chapter. If you or your family love homemade pizza, consider getting a bread machine so you can make it easily and more often. For more about bread machines see pages 41 to 42.

French Drip Coffee

Gluten-Free

The 1973 Joy of Cooking *says, "Coffee has always thrived on adversity – just as people in adversity have thrived on coffee." Unless you must avoid coffee for health reasons, you don't have to give it up now. Just make it inexpensively at home.*

2 level measuring tablespoons drip-grind coffee
1 cup boiling water

Place a filter in the top of your drip coffee-making system. Add the coffee to the filter. (You can do this in the evening if you will be in a rush the next morning). Bring the water to a boil and pour it into the filter. If there is more water than room in the filter, add the water a little at a time. Let the water drip through completely and enjoy! You may double this recipe to make enough coffee for a 16-ounce travel mug such as the Melitta Ready-Set-Joe Travel Mug and Cone system.

Notes about French drip coffee: I suspect that the reason that manually-made drip coffee is called "French drip" is because the French expect excellence in coffee and, in my opinion, this method makes the best tasting coffee. Unlike automatic coffee makers, there is no build up of hard water scum. The temperature is never too hot (which can be a problem with percolators) causing bitterness. When you make coffee with this method, the result is dependent only on the quality of the coffee itself. If you are devoted to Starbucks™, buy their coffee to use in this recipe. To add variety to your morning brew, shop around to find your favorite bulk coffees, purchase them in small quantities, and grind them at the store or at home. An Internet source estimates that a large mug of homemade French drip coffee costs less than 50 cents per day which in a year's time will save you several hundred dollars over a daily stop at the coffee shop.

Tips for best flavor: Avoid using coffee that has been ground in the distant past. Store ground coffee in an airtight container such as a nut butter jar with rubber sealing material around the edge of the lid. If you will not be using ground coffee quickly, store it in the freezer. Use fresh soft (not softened) water. If the water is hard in your area, use bottled water. If you must re-heat your coffee, do it very carefully and do not let it boil or it will become bitter.

Fruit Juice Soda

Gluten-Free

This drink recipe lets you save money while avoiding the sugar, corn sweetener or artificial sweeteners, phosphates, and caffeine found in most soft drinks.

¼ cup of any sugar-free frozen fruit juice concentrate, thawed, such as
        apple, pineapple, grape, white grape, or a fruit blend
¾ cup chilled carbonated water
A few ice cubes.

Stir together all of the ingredients in a tall glass. Add a straw and enjoy. Makes one serving.

Good and Healthy Popcorn

Gluten-Free

Make your own popcorn using this recipe and you will save money while you control the amount and type of fat you consume. Even organic or "natural" microwave popcorn often contains unhealthy types of fat. This is the way popcorn was when I was a kid – delicious!

> 2 tablespoons oil
> ⅓ cup unpopped popcorn
> ⅛ teaspoon salt, or to taste
> Melted butter (optional)

Put the oil in a 3 quart or slightly larger saucepan. Add three kernels of popcorn to the pan and heat it over medium heat on your stove. For safety's sake, stay close by and watch the pan carefully. In a minute or two, you will hear the three kernels of popcorn pop. Immediately add the rest of the popcorn to the pan. Move the pan back and forth on the burner while the popcorn pops. When the popping slows down and nearly stops, remove the pan from the stove. Pour the popcorn into a bowl. Sprinkle it with salt and toss it with melted butter if desired. This makes a great, nutritious, very healthy snack. If your family wants to snack routinely, make a double batch using a larger pan and leave it out in a bowl on your kitchen counter. Makes 2 to 2½ quarts of popcorn.

Sweet 'n Nutty Popcorn

Gluten-Free

This homemade caramelcorn is sweetened with healthy sweeteners and is much more economical than similar store-bought snacks.

> 2 to 2½ quarts air-popped popcorn or one batch of popcorn, above
> 1 cup slivered almonds or chopped nuts of any kind
> ¼ cup (½ stick) of butter, ghee, goat butter, or Earth Balance™ margarine
> ½ cup agave, honey, or Fruit Sweet™
> ½ teaspoon salt (optional – use only if you use unsalted butter or ghee)
> 1 teaspoon vanilla extract, almond flavoring, orange flavoring, or
>   flavoring of your choice (optional)
> ¼ teaspoon baking soda

Pop the popcorn and put it in a large bowl with the nuts. In a saucepan, combine the butter or margarine, sweetener, and salt. Use the salt only if you use unsalted butter or ghee. Heat the mixture over medium heat until it begins to bubble. Reduce the heat to low and let it simmer for 5 minutes. While it is cooking, preheat your oven to 250°F. Remove the pan from the stove when the simmering time is completed. Stir in the flavoring thoroughly. Then stir in the baking soda thoroughly. The liquid will become a very fine foam. Pour the liquid over the popcorn and nuts and stir thoroughly to coat the popcorn and nuts uniformly. Put the popcorn mixture in a 13 inch by 9 inch cake pan, a jelly roll pan, or two 8 or 9 inch cake pans. Bake the popcorn for 30 minutes, stirring it every 10 minutes. Remove it from the oven and allow it to cool. Stir it a few times while it is cooling to break it up. When it is completely cooled, store it in a tightly covered container or plastic bag. Makes 4 to 8 servings.

Power Snack Cookies

Gluten-Free IF
made with amaranth flour

This delicious alternative to energy bars is gluten-free and high in protein when made with amaranth flour. My husband, a wheat-eater who does not like peanut butter cookies, loves these cookies made with cashew butter and amaranth flour.

2 cups rye flour OR 1½ cups amaranth flour plus ½ cup arrowroot or
    tapioca starch
½ teaspoon baking soda
⅛ teaspoon unbuffered vitamin C powder
⅔ cup cashew butter or natural* peanut butter
¼ cup oil
¾ cup agave or maple syrup
1 teaspoon vanilla (optional)

Preheat your oven to 400°F. If you are using the agave, line your baking sheets with parchment paper for easiest cookie removal or lightly oil the baking sheets.

Combine the flour(s), baking soda, and vitamin C powder in a large bowl. In a small bowl, thoroughly mix together the nut butter, oil, agave or maple syrup, and vanilla. (A hand blender is helpful for thorough mixing especially if the nut butter is fairly solid from having been refrigerated). Stir and mash the nut butter mixture into the dry ingredients. Drop the dough by heaping teaspoonfuls onto baking sheets. Use an oiled fork to flatten the balls of dough, making an "X" on the top of them with the fork tines. Bake the cookies for 8 to 10 minutes, or until they are golden brown. Makes about 3 dozen cookies.

Note on peanut butter: Use peanut butter which contains only peanuts and salt (usually called natural peanut butter) and does not contain hydrogenated fats or added sweeteners.

Pizza

Gluten-Free IF
made with rice or buckwheat crust

Homemade pizza is really not all that difficult to make especially if you use a bread machine to make the dough. For many more varieties of dough including yeast-free dough, see The Ultimate Food Allergy Cookbook and Survival Guide *as described on the last pages of this book.*

> 1 batch pizza dough, pages 179 to 180, or 1 batch of dough for Buckwheat "Rye" Bread, page 148, made without the caraway seed and rye flavor
> ½ batch of pizza sauce, page 178
> 3 to 4 ounces low fat or part-skim mozzarella cheese or other type of cheese which you tolerate
> 2 tablespoons grated Romano cheese, Parmesan cheese, or all-sheep milk Romano cheese (optional – if tolerated)
> ½ to 1 cup chopped vegetables such as green peppers, olives, etc.
> 2 ounces cooked meat such as cooked lean ground beef or buffalo, pepperoni, etc. (optional – if tolerated)

Begin making the pizza dough as directed in the recipe. If you make the buckwheat dough, omit the rye flavor and caraway seeds. While the dough is rising, make the pizza sauce and prepare the baking pan.

For the spelt pizza, very lightly oil a baking sheet or 12 inch pizza pan by putting a teaspoon or less of oil on a paper towel and rubbing the paper towel on the baking sheet or all around the bottom and edges of the pizza pan. Turn the dough out onto your bread board or kitchen counter. The oil on the dough should be sufficient to keep it from sticking to the bread board counter. Stretch or roll it out into a 12-inch circle. Transfer the dough to the baking sheet or pizza pan. You may have to push and stretch it with your hands to get it to fit all the way to the edges of the pizza pan.

For the rice or buckwheat pizza, while the dough is resting for 5 minutes after the final beating or at the end of the bread machine dough cycle, oil and flour a 12-inch pizza pan. Coat the inside of the pan with the kind of flour you used in the dough. Let the dough rest for about 5 minutes after the last beating and then transfer it to the prepared pan. Oil your fingers and use them to spread the dough evenly to the edges of the pan.

If you like thin crust pizza, preheat your oven, top the dough immediately, and bake it as directed in the next paragraph. If you prefer a thick crust pizza, place the pizza in a pre-warmed oven (see the third paragraph on page 179) or in a warm spot in your kitchen and let the dough rise for about 5 to 10 minutes for gluten-free rice or buckwheat dough or about 10 to 15 minutes for spelt dough, or until it begins to puff up slightly. Remove the pizza from the oven.

Preheat your oven to 400°F. While the oven is heating, spread the pizza with sauce for one pizza (half of what you made in the recipe below) and the desired toppings. Bake it for 20 to 25 minutes or until the edge is golden brown. Makes one 12 inch pizza.

Pizza Sauce

Gluten-Free

Making this sauce is a snap; I make a quadruple batch and freeze it for future use.

    1 6 ounce can tomato paste
    1 8 ounce can tomato sauce
    ⅓ cup water
    1 teaspoon dry oregano
    ½ teaspoon dry thyme
    ½ teaspoon dry sweet basil
    1 tablespoon olive oil (optional)

Combine all the sauce ingredients in a saucepan and heat on medium heat until the sauce begins to boil. Reduce the heat to low and simmer the sauce for 30 to 45 minutes or until it become thicker, stirring every ten minutes to keep the sauce from sticking to the bottom of the pan. This makes enough sauce for two pizzas. You can either freeze half of the sauce for future use or double the amounts of dough and toppings you use and have two pizzas. If you do not eat both pizzas, the leftover pizza will freeze well.

White Spelt Pizza Dough

⅔ cup water at about 115°F

2½ tablespoons apple juice concentrate, thawed, or 1 tablespoon agave,
Fruit Sweet™ or honey plus 1½ tablespoons water

1 tablespoon oil

½ teaspoon salt

2¼ to 2½ cups white spelt flour

1¼ teaspoons active dry or quick rise yeast

To make this dough in a bread machine, add the ingredients to the pan in the order listed using the smaller amount of flour and active dry yeast. Start the dough cycle. Check the dough after several minutes of kneading and adjust the consistency of the dough by adding more flour if needed.

To make this dough using a mixer, follow the procedure on pages 150 to 151.

To make the dough by hand, mix together the water and sweetener in a large bowl. Sprinkle the surface of the liquid with the yeast, then stir the yeast into the liquid. Allow it to stand for about 10 minutes until it begins to get foamy. Stir in the oil, salt, and about half of the flour. Add the remaining flour a little at a time until you've added as much of the flour as you can stir in by hand. Spread a little of the remaining flour on a bread board or your kitchen counter. Put the dough on the bread board or counter and knead in as much of the remaining flour as it takes to make a soft yet smooth and elastic dough. Knead the dough for 10 minutes.

While you are kneading the dough, unless you have a very cozy (85 to 90°F) corner in your kitchen, begin to prepare your oven to be a rising spot for the dough. If you have a gas oven, the pilot light will probably keep the oven at just about the right temperature, 85 to 90°F. If you have an electric oven, turn it on to 350°F and let it preheat. Turn it off, open the oven, and let it cool for 8 to 10 minutes until the temperature inside the oven is about 85 to 90°F. Then close the oven door.

When the handmade or mixer-made dough is well kneaded, wash out the mixing bowl you used to make it and dry it. Rub the inside of the bowl generously with oil. Put the dough into the bowl and turn it over so the top side of the dough is also oiled. Cover the dough with plastic wrap. Place the bowl in your pre-warmed oven or a warm spot in your kitchen and let it rise until doubled. This will take about an hour if you used active dry yeast or about 40 minutes if you used quick rise yeast. Then punch the dough down by plunging your fist into the middle of it. Let it rest for about five minutes before shaping it into a pizza. If you made your dough in a bread machine, let it rest for about five minutes after the dough cycle is finished if there was a stir down at the end of the cycle. Use this dough to make one pizza as directed on pages 177 to 178.

If you have a large 2-pound bread machine, you can use it to make a double batch of this dough for two pizzas. If it is not mixing efficiently at the beginning of the dough cycle, help mix the dough with a narrow rubber spatula. The Zojirushi BBCC-X20 will mix a double batch without assistance; a double batch can be set up with the delayed start timer and produce great dough while you are away. This recipe can also be doubled to yield two pizzas if you make it by hand or using a mixer.

Leftover homemade pizza freezes well for a future meal. To reheat it, put it in the pizza pan, cover it with foil, and bake it at 375°F for 20-30 minutes. (The baking time depends on how close to thawed the pizza is when you put it in the oven). Touch the top of the pizza with your hand at about 15 minutes into the baking time and then every 5 minutes. Bake it until it just becomes hot.

Rice Pizza Dough

Gluten-Free

4 large or 3 extra-large eggs (enough to yield ¾ cup of slightly beaten egg)
        at room temperature
¼ cup apple juice, thawed
½ cup water at about 115°F
2 tablespoons oil
1 teaspoon salt
2 cups brown or white rice flour
⅓ cup potato flour
⅓ cup tapioca starch or arrowroot
4 teaspoons guar gum
⅛ teaspoon unbuffered vitamin C powder
1 package (2¼ teaspoons) active dry or quick-rise yeast
Additional rice flour to coat the pan

Remove the eggs from the refrigerator and allow them to warm to room temperature. If you forget to take them out of the refrigerator ahead, put them in a bowl of warm water for about 5 minutes while you are gathering the other ingredients.

To make this dough in a bread machine, use the active dry yeast rather than quick-rise yeast and stir the guar gum into the rice flour. Add the ingredients (except the additional flour to coat the pan) to the bread machine pan in the order listed and start the dough cycle.

To make this dough with a mixer, put the 2 cups of rice flour, potato flour, arrowroot or tapioca starch, yeast, guar gum, vitamin C, and salt in a large mixer bowl. Mix on low speed for about 30 seconds. In a small saucepan, warm the juice, water and oil to 115-120°F. (Measure the temperature with a yeast thermometer). Do not warm the eggs. With the mixer running on low speed, add the liquids to the dry ingredients in a slow stream. Beat the eggs slightly, measure out ¾ cup of beaten egg, and add them to the bowl with the mixer running. Continue mixing until the dry and liquid ingredients are thoroughly mixed. Beat the dough on medium speed for 3 minutes. Scrape the dough from the beaters and the sides of the bowl into the bottom of the bowl. Cover the bowl, put it in a warm (85°F to 90°F) place and let the dough rise for 1 to 1½ hours or until double in volume. (See the third paragraph on page 179 for how to use your oven as a cozy rising place). Beat the dough again for three minutes at medium speed. Let it rest for about 5 minutes. While it is resting, oil a 12-inch pizza pan and coat the inside of it generously with additional rice flour. Put the dough into the prepared pan and stretch it out to fill the pan. Top it with pizza toppings and bake it as directed in the pizza recipe on page 178.

If made with a mixer, you can double this recipe to yield two pizzas and freeze the leftover pizza for a future meal. See the previous recipe for directions on reheating leftover pizza.

Designer GORP

Gluten-Free

*Use your imagination to make this an original take-off on **Good Old Raisins and Peanuts**. Make it with almonds, pumpkin seeds, and sunflower seeds for a good serving of essential fatty acids and you will get maximum nutrition for your money.*

> 2 cups of nuts and seeds of two or three different kinds (i.e. peanuts and sunflower seeds, almonds and cashews, or pumpkin seeds, sunflower seeds and almonds)
> 1½ cups of raisins or other small or diced dried fruit
> 1 cup of grain-sweetened or regular chocolate chips or carob chips (optional)

Mix all of the ingredients together in a plastic bag. Take the bag along with you for a healthy energizing snack away from home. Makes about 3½ to 4½ cups of snack mix.

Using Commercially Prepared Foods

Commercially prepared foods, although more expensive than homemade, can be great savers of kitchen time for those on allergy and celiac diets. However, commercial foods may contain hidden allergens. **You MUST READ LABELS** very carefully to determine which foods you can use. Finding safe commercially prepared foods can be challenging, but it is not impossible.

Allergenic foods often appear on ingredient lists in disguise. For instance, if the ingredient list contains maltodextrin, people who are allergic to corn should not eat that food. A list of derivatives of common allergenic foods which can appear as disguised or hidden allergenic ingredients is below. Although I have attempted to make it complete, **this list may not be exhaustive;** other ingredients might be derived from your problem foods which are not listed below. Prepared foods which in their usual form contain a certain allergen also are included in this list. For example, bread is on the list as a source of wheat. However, not all bread is made with wheat; there are a large number of gluten-and wheat free breads on the market. (See pages 188 to 189). You must read the labels of all foods purchased to see if you can or cannot eat them.

Hidden Allergens and Food Derivatives to Avoid in Commercially Prepared Foods and Common Problem Foods and Products

WHEAT:

Adhesive stamps and envelopes. Do not lick them; apply water with a sponge instead.

Alcoholic beverages made from grains such as beer, whiskey, gin, and some vodka

Bulgur

Candy – some. Wheat flour may be used for dusting during processing.

Cooking oil spray – some

Couscous

Dextrin – some

Flavorings or extracts – Some contain grain-source alcohol.

Flour, durum flour, graham flour, gluten flour, wheat flour, semolina flour

Gluten

Grain-based coffee substitutes such as Postum™

Hydrolyzed vegetable protein (HVP) or hydrolyzed plant protein (HPP
– some

Imitation seafood or sirimi. Some contain wheat starch as a binder.

Medications, prescription or over-the-counter. Some use wheat starch as a
binder or filler.

Modified food starch or modified starch – some

Monosodium glutamate (MSG)

Pasta, including those such as Jerusalem artichoke pasta made with semolina
flour. Wheat and gluten-free types of pasta are listed in the next chapter.

Poultry, self-basting – some

Processed and canned meats – some

Wheat germ, bran, or berries, cracked wheat

Wheat products such as bread, crackers, etc.

White (grain) vinegar

GLUTEN:

**All of the items listed above and on the previous page under "Wheat"
plus:**

Alcoholic spirits – some. Canadian celiac groups say that distillation prevents
gluten from entering the final product; American groups are not sure. Ask
your doctor.

Caramel coloring, if imported source

Coffee – some. Flavored coffees may contain gluten. Freeze-dried coffee is the
safest. Consult the manufacturer.

Grains, some in addition to wheat such as rye, barley, spelt, kamut and
triticale. Oats might or might not be allowed; ask your doctor.

Herbal teas – A few contain malt.

Malt, malt flavoring, malt vinegar

Rice syrup – some

Soy sauce – some

Vegetable gum, vegetable protein – some

Vinegar – some which are made from grain. Canadian celiac groups say that
distillation prevents gluten from entering the final product; American
groups are not sure. Ask your doctor.

MILK:

Casein, sodium caseinate, or caseinate

Curds

Hydrolyzed vegetable protein (HVP) or hydrolyzed plant protein (HPP)
— some

Lactalbumin

Lactoglobulin

Lactose

Medications, prescription or over-the-counter. Some use lactose as a filler.

Milk products such as butter, cheese, cream, etc.

Powdered, evaporated, or condensed milk

Processed and canned meats – some

Whey

EGGS:

Albumin

Egg pasta

Egg products such as powdered or dried egg, egg yolk, or egg white

Egg substitutes such as EggBeaters™

Globulin

Meringue

Ovomucoid

Ovomucin

Ovovitellin or vitellin

Sauces such as mayonnaise, hollandaise, or tartar sauce

Wine – Some wines may be clarified with egg white.

CORN:

Adhesive stamps and envelopes. Do not lick them; apply water with a sponge
instead.

Alcoholic beverages – some, especially sweet wines

Baking powder – most contain cornstarch

Caramel coloring – some

Corn flour, cornmeal, corn oil, corn syrup, corn sweetener

Cornstarch – often used as a filler in supplements and medications

Dextrose

Dextrin – some

Egg substitutes such as EggBeaters™ might contain maltodextrin, etc.

Flavorings such as vanilla may contain corn syrup

Fructose, which is also called levulose – some

Glucose – some

Grits

Hominy

Hydrolyzed vegetable protein (HVP) or hydrolyzed plant protein (HPP)
    – some

Imitation seafood or sirimi. Some contain cornstarch as a binder.

Instant tea – some

Maltodextrin

Medications, prescription or over-the-counter. Some use cornstarch as a
    binder or filler.

Modified food starch, food starch

Paper and plastic items – Some plastic wraps and plastic or paper cups and
    plates may be coated with corn oil.

Poultry, self-basting – some

Powdered sugar (contains cornstarch)

Salt – Some contain dextrose to prevent caking.

Sugar alcohols such as sorbitol, xylitol, maltitol, etc. are usually made from
    corn.

Vitamin C – most. Some brands labeled as "synthetic" are actually
    manufactured from corn. Allergy Research Group sells cassava-source
    vitamin C. See "Sources," page 211 for ordering information.

Xanthum gum – May be produced using a corn-source base.

SOY:

Cooking oil spray – some

Hydrolyzed vegetable protein (HVP) or hydrolyzed plant protein (HPP)
    – some

Lecithin

Margarine – Most margarine contains soy oil or lecithin

Miso

Processed meats – some

Shortening – most

(SOY, continued)

Soy flour, soy oil, soy meal, soy milk
Tamari, soy sauce, worcestershire sauce
Tempeh
Textured vegetable protein (TVP)
Tofu

YEAST:

All alcoholic beverages
Black (fermented) teas
Cheese
Enriched grain products – Most are enriched with vitamins from yeast.
Malted products
Soft drinks which may contain fermented products such as root beer and
    ginger ale
Soy sauce and condiments which contain soy sauce
Vinegar (all kinds) and condiments which contain vinegar, such as mustard,
    pickles, etc.
Vitamins and vitamin enriched processed foods – some. Hypoallergenic
    vitamins may be yeast-free.
Yeast breads. Sourdough is NOT yeast-free, but contains "wild" yeasts which
    some yeast sensitive people can tolerate.
Other foods: If your doctor puts you on a yeast-free diet, he or she may also
    advise you to avoid leftovers, fruit juices, mushrooms, dried fruits and
    spices, all types of tea, sugar, and other foods which may aggravate
    candidiasis.

Special Diet Resources
Foods and Their Producers

This chapter contains a list of some commercially made foods that you might be able to use on your diet. **READ THE LABELS** on these items before you purchase them; manufacturers change ingredients often and may have changed them since the time of this writing. Large health food stores carry many of the items listed. Contact information is given for each company to help your health food store find foods they do not carry. Some of the companies listed welcome individual orders. Many of them make products in addition to those listed below which you also may be able to use. Visit the company websites listed below for up-to-date information about all of their products.

This list contains only relatively "clean" foods and therefore is not exhaustive. Many good products can be found that eliminate some problem foods but contain several other common allergens; these are usually not listed below.

This book contains comments about what I can buy at *my* health food store. After talking to people from all over the country, I concluded that the store where I shop, Vitamin Cottage Natural Grocers, is much better for people with allergies and celiac disease than many health food stores. Therefore, the first listing below is for the Vitamin Cottage website. They will ship the products listed on their website anywhere in the country, so if you can afford to pay for shipping on something you need badly but cannot get locally, try the Vitamin Cottage website.

THE VITAMIN COTTAGE

Almost everything you need in one place.

Vitamin Cottage Natural Grocers
12612 W. Alameda Parkway
Lakewood, CO 80228
(800) 817-9415 or 303-986-4600
email: CustomerService@VitaminCottage.com
http://naturalgrocers.com/
  Shop by diet page: http://naturalgrocers.com/shop-by-diet.html

BREADS

Most of the breads below are sourdough breads. They contain wild yeast from the air even though it may not be listed as an ingredient.

Food For Life White Rice Bread: White rice flour, water, honey, soy oil, guar gum, xanthum gum, cellulose, yeast, sea salt

Food for Life Baking Company, Inc.
P.O. Box 1434
Corona, CA 92878
(800) 797-5090 or (951) 279-5090
www.foodforlife.com

French Meadow Spelt Bread: Spelt, water, sea salt
French Meadow Rye Bread: Rye, water, sea salt

French Meadow Bakery
2610 Lyndale Avenue South
Minneapolis, MN 55408
1-877-NOYEAST or (612) 870-4740
www.frenchmeadow.com

Nokomis Bakery Spelt and Kamut Sourdough Breads

Nokomis Bakery
2463 County Road ES
East Troy, WI 53120
(800) 367-0358
www.nokomisbakery.com

Pacific Bakery Kamut Bread: Organic kamut, water, sea salt
Pacific Bakery Spelt Bread: Spelt, water, sea salt

Pacific Bakery
P.O. Box 950
Oceanside, California 92049
(760) 757-6020
www,pacificbakery.com

Rudi's Spelt Bread: Organic spelt flour, water, honey, yeast, canola oil, salt, lecithin

Rudi's Organic Bakery
3300 Walnut, Unit C
Boulder, CO 80301
(877) 293-0876 or (303) 447-0495
www.rudisbakery.com

Rudolph's 100% Rye Bread: Organic rye flour, water, sourdough culture, salt

Rudolph's Specialty Bakeries Ltd.
390 Alliance Avenue
Toronto, Ontario, Canada M6N 2H8
(416) 763-4315
www.rudolphsbreads.com

TORTILLAS AND FLATBREADS

AMARANTH

Amaranth Flatbread: amaranth flour, water, garbanzo flour, safflower oil, sea salt

Nu-World Amaranth, Inc.
P.O. Box 2202
Naperville, IL 60567
(630) 369-6819
www.nuworldfoods.com

RICE

Food for Life Brown Rice Tortillas: Whole grain brown rice flour, filtered water, tapioca flour, safflower oil, rice bran, vegetable gum (xanthum, cellulose), sea salt.

Food for Life Baking Company, Inc.
P.O. Box 1434
Corona, CA 92878
(800) 797-5090 or (951) 279-5090
www.foodforlife.com

HEMP

French Meadow Gluten-Free Healthy Hemp Tortillas: Organic sunflower seed, filtered water, organic flaxseed, organic pumpkin seed, organic hemp flour, organic hemp seed, organic amaranth flour, organic unrefined sunflower oil, organic sesame seed, organic arrowroot, unrefined sea salt, guar gum, organic nutmeg, non-aluminum baking powder, organic cayenne.

French Meadow Bakery
2610 Lyndale Avenue South
Minneapolis, MN 55408
1-877-NOYEAST or (612) 870-4740
www.frenchmeadow.com

SPELT

Rudi's Organic Spelt or Whole Spelt Tortillas: Organic spelt flour (or whole spelt flour), organic palm fruit shortening, cultured spelt flour, organic honey, sea salt, apple cider vinegar, cream of tartar, organic oat fiber, natural enzymes, ascorbic acid, sodium bicarbonate. (These are not yeast-free because of the cultured spelt flour and vinegar).

Rudi's Organic Bakery
3300 Walnut, Unit C
Boulder, CO 80301
(877) 293-0876 or (303) 447-0495
www.rudisbakery.com

CRACKERS

RICE CAKES, many brands: Watch out for other grains, popcorn, cheese, and sweeteners that may be included in the ingredients.

RICE CRACKERS

Edward & Sons Brown Rice Snaps: Plain flavor ingredients: Organic brown rice flour, organic white rice flour. (A variety of flavors is available).

Edward & Sons Trading Company
P.O. Box 1326
Carpenteria, CA 93014
(805) 684-8500
www.edwardandsons.com

Hol-Grain Brown Rice Crackers: Brown rice, salt

Conrad Rice Mill, Inc.
P.O. Box 10640
New Iberia, LA 70560
(800) 551-3245 or (337) 364-7242
www.conradricemill.com

Westbrae Natural Unsalted Brown Rice Wafers: Brown rice, sesame seeds

Westbrae Natural Foods
The Hain Celestial Group, Inc.
4600 Sleepytime Drive
Boulder, CO 80301
(800) 434-4246
www.westbrae.com

RICE PLUS NUT CRACKERS

Blue Diamond Nut Thins, Pecan flavor: Rice flour, pecan meal, potato starch, safflower oil, salt, natural pecan flavor, natural butter flavor (contains milk).

Blue Diamond Growers
1802 C Street
P.O. Box 1768
Sacramento CA, 95811
(916) 442-0771
www.bluediamond.com

(Blue Diamond Crackers, continued)

Blue Diamond makes other varieties of crackers. The Smokehouse Almond variety contains torula yeast and soy. The Country Ranch variety contains several milk products including buttermilk, sour cream, and whey.

RYE CRACKERS

RyVita Tasty Dark Rye or Tasty Light Rye Crackers: Whole grain rye, salt
(These crackers are widely available in health food stores).

InterNatural Foods, LLC.
15 Prospect Street
Paramus, NJ 07652
(201) 909-0808
www.internaturalfoods.com/Ryvita/Ryvita.html

Wasa Original Crispbread: Light Rye variety: whole grain rye flour, water, salt
(These crackers are widely available in health food stores).

GermanDeli.com
2890 Market Loop
Southlake, TX 76092
(877) GERMANY
www.germandeli.com/wasacrispbread.html

COOKIES, GLUTEN-FREE

Nana's Single-Serve Cookies: Several of the varieties are gluten-, egg-, and dairy free. They are made with rice and fruit sweetened. The price is about $1.50 for a single large cookie.

Nana's Cookie Company
4901 Morena Blvd., Suite 401
San Diego, CA 92117
(800) 826-7534
www.healthycrowd.com

Jennie's Coconut Macaroons: Coconut, honey, egg whites

Red Mill Farms, Inc.
209 South 5th Street
Brooklyn, NY 11211
(888) 294-1164
www.jennies-macaroons.com

CEREALS, HOT

Single rolled grains such as oatmeal from the health food store are a good choice for making hot cereal. Many packaged hot cereals contain mixed grains. The packaged hot cereals listed below contain a single grain.

Lundberg Hot & Creamy Rice Cereal: Oven-roasted organic whole grain California rice

Lundberg Family Farms
5370 Church Street
Richvale, CA 95974
(530) 882-4551
www.lundberg.com

Arrowhead Mills Rice and Shine: Organic brown rice grits

Arrowhead Mills
The Hain Celestial Group, Inc.
4600 Sleepytime Drive
Boulder, CO 80301
(800) 434-4246
www.hain-celestial.com

Pocono Cream of Buckwheat: 100% Buckwheat

Birkett Mills
163 Main Street
Penn Yan, NY 14527
(315) 536-3311
www.thebirkettmills.com

CEREALS, COLD

Except for puffed grains, most cold cereals are made from several grains. A few types of cold cereals that contain more simple ingredients are listed here.

Puffed Amaranth: Amaranth only

Nu-World Amaranth, Inc.
P.O. Box 2202
Naperville, IL 60567
(630) 369-6819
www.nuworldfoods.com

Arrowhead Mills Puffed Rice: Brown rice only
Arrowhead Mills Puffed Millet: Millet only
Arrowhead Mills Organic Spelt Flakes: Spelt, apple, pear and peach juice concentrates, sea salt, vitamin C, vitamin E

Arrowhead Mills
The Hain Celestial Group, Inc.
4600 Sleepytime Drive
Boulder, CO 80301
(800) 434-4246
www.hain-celestial.com

Barbara's Brown Rice Crisps: Brown rice, pineapple juice concentrate, pear juice concentrate, peach juice concentrate, sea salt
Barbara's Breakfast O's: Whole oat flour, brown rice flour, pineapple juice concentrate, pear juice concentrate, oat bran, peach juice concentrate, sea salt.

Barbara's Bakery, Inc.
3900 Cypress Drive
Petaluma, CA 94954
(707) 765-2273
www.barbarasbakery.com

Erewhon Kamut Flakes: Kamut, pear juice concentrate, sea salt
Erewhon Crispy Brown Rice Cereal (NOT gluten-free): Brown rice, barley malt, sea salt (also comes salt-free)

Erewhon Cereals
U.S. Mills, Inc.
200 Reservoir Street
Needham, MA 02494-3146
(781) 444-0440
www.usmillsinc.com

GLUTEN-FREE BAKING MIXES

Because of the great number of mixes each of these companies makes, only general comments about the brand of mixes are given rather than full ingredient lists for each mix. If you wish to purchase an assortment of mixes, at the time of this writing these mixes are available from the Vitamin Cottage website (http://naturalgrocers.com/). For more information about the ingredients in each mix, contact the manufacturer or visit Vitamin Cottage website, shop by brand or by diet, find the mix, and click on "back of the bag" to see the ingredient list.

CASSAVA-BASED MIXES

Chebe™ Bread Mixes – Several varieties including cheese bread mix, all purpose bread mix, focaccia mix, pizza crust mix, garlic-onion bread sticks, and cinnamon roll-up mix. All of the mixes require the addition of eggs; some also require milk products.

Chebe™ Bread Products
1840 Lundberg Drive
Spirit Lake, IA 51360
(800) 217-9510
http://chebe.com/

RICE-BASED MIXES

1-2-3 Gluten Free Mixes: Although all of these mixes are rice-based, if you can have rice, they are a good choice because many of them are corn-, milk-, egg-, and soy-free.

1-2-3 Gluten Free Inc.
5145 Penton Road
Pittsburgh, PA 15213
(843) 768-7231
www.123glutenfree.com

Namaste Baking Mixes: These rice-based mixes are usually corn-free. All of the mixes except for the pizza crust mix call for the addition of eggs. Some of the mixes are sugar free.

Namaste Foods, LLC
P.O. Box 3133
Coeur d'Alene, ID 83816
(866) 258-9493 or (208) 772-6325
www.namastefoods.com

Pamela's Baking Mixes: These rice-based mixes seem heavy on sugar, honey, and molasses and many of the mixes contain corn, butter, or other allergens, but a celiac friend raves about how delicious they are, so they are included in this list.

Pamela's Products, Inc.
200 Clara Avenue
Ukiah, CA 95482
Phone 707-462-6605
www.pamelasproducts.com

SORGHUM, BEAN, ETC.-BASED MIXES

The following companies make some rice-free mixes as well as rice-based mixes.

Authentic Foods Baking Mixes: Authentic Foods was the first company to make sorghum easily available and makes some rice-free mixes (such as Bette's Four Flour

Blend) as well as rice-containing mixes. Their baking mixes include Pancake and Baking Mix, Bread Mix Homestyle, Falafel Mix, Pizza Crust Mix, Cinnamon Bread Mix, Vanilla, Chocolate, and Lemon Cake Mixes, and Blueberry and Chocolate Chip Muffin Mixes.

Authentic Foods
1850 W. 168th Street, Suite B
Gardena, CA 90247
(800) 806-4737 or (310) 366-7612
www.authenticfoods.com

Bob's Red Mill Baking Mixes: Some of Bob's mixes are based on a blend of several flours including sorghum, garbanzo, fava, potato, tapioca, and in many cases also contain corn.

Bob's Red Mill Natural Foods Inc.
5209 S.E. International Way
Milwaukie, OR 97222
(800) 349-2173 or (503) 654-3215
www.bobsredmill.com

PASTA

Read pasta labels carefully to be sure that they only contain the grains you can eat. Most buckwheat (soba) pasta contains wheat, Jerusalem artichoke pasta contains semolina, which is a variety of wheat, and wheat-free quinoa pasta contains corn.

BUCKWHEAT

Eden 100% Soba Japanese Buckwheat Pasta: Buckwheat only.

Eden Foods, Inc.
701 Tecumseh Road
Clinton, MI 49236
(888) 424-EDEN (3336) or (517) 456-7424
www.edenfoods.com

BEAN

Eden Mung Bean Pasta: Bean starch only

Eden Foods, Inc.
701 Tecumseh Road
Clinton, MI 49236
(888) 424-EDEN (3336) or (517) 456-7424
www.edenfoods.com

CORN

Westbrae Natural Corn Pasta: Corn flour only

Westbrae Natural Foods
The Hain Celestial Group, Inc.
4600 Sleepytime Drive
Boulder, CO 80301
(800) 434-4246
www.westbrae.com

DeBole's Corn Spaghetti and Elbow Macaroni: Yellow corn meal, yellow corn flour

DeBole's Nutritional Foods
The Hain Celestial Group, Inc.
4600 Sleepytime Drive
Boulder, CO 80301
(800) 434-4246
www.hain-celestial.com

KAMUT AND RYE (Contain gluten)

Eden Kamut or Rye Pasta: Whole grain kamut flour only or whole grain rye flour only

Eden Foods, Inc.
701 Tecumseh Road
Clinton, MI 49236
(888) 424-EDEN (3336) or (517) 456-7424
www.edenfoods.com

QUINOA

Quinoa Pasta: Quinoa flour, corn flour

The Quinoa Corporation
Post Office Box 279
Gardena, CA. 90248
(310) 217-8125
www.quinoa.net

RICE

DeBole's No-boil Rice Lasagne, Spaghetti, and Fettuccini, Penne, and Spirals:
Rice flour, rice bran extract

DeBole's Nutritional Foods
The Hain Celestial Group, Inc.
4600 Sleepytime Drive
Boulder, CO 80301
(800) 434-4246
www.hain-celestial.com

Ener-G Rice Macaroni, Lasagne, Spaghetti, or Shells: Rice flour, water

Ener-G Foods, Inc.
P. O. Box 84487
Seattle, WA 98124
(800) 331-5222 or (206) 767-6660
www.ener-g.com

SPELT

Vita-Spelt Spaghetti, Shells, Medium Shells, Elbow Macaroni, Rotini, Lasagne, and Angel Hair: spelt flour, water; **Egg Noodles:** spelt flour, egg, water

Purity Foods, Inc.
2871 W. Jolly Road
Okemos, MI 48864
(517) 351-9231
www.purityfoods.com

MEATS

Unprocessed meats are naturally gluten-free. However, if you have a craving for a hot dog or lunch meat, try Shelton's gluten-free franks and bologna. If you can eat turkey but not the corn- or wheat- derived additives and flavorings, try Shelton's frozen ground turkey.

Shelton's Uncured Chicken or Turkey Franks or Bologna: Mechanically separated chicken or turkey, water, potato starch, sea salt, ground mustard seed, spices.
Shelton's Ground Free Range Turkey: Free range turkey

Shelton's Poultry, Inc.
204 N. Loranne
Pomona, CA 91767
(800) 541-1833 or (909) 623-4361
www.sheltons.com

FRUIT AND VEGETABLE PRODUCTS

CANNED BEANS

Westbrae Natural Organic Cooked Beans (black beans, kidney beans, great northern beans, red beans, pinto beans, garbanzo beans, soybeans, lentils, split peas): Water, organic cooked beans (of the specified type), sea salt.

Westbrae Natural Foods
The Hain Celestial Group, Inc.
4600 Sleepytime Drive
Boulder, CO 80301
(800) 434-4246
www.westbrae.com

CANNED FRUITS AND VEGETABLES

Read the labels carefully because some brands of organic "health food" veg-etables contain sugar or organic cane juice.

S & W water-packed fruits and vegetables: contain the specified fruit or vegetable and water

S & W Fine Foods, Inc.
P.O. Box 193575
San Francisco, CA 94119-3575
(800) 252-7033
www.swfinefoods.com

Santa Cruz Organic Applesauce: organic apples only

Santa Cruz Naturals, Inc.
P.O. Box 369
Chico, CA 95927
(530) 899-5010
www.scojuice.com

FROZEN FRUITS AND VEGETABLES

Cascadian Farms Organic Frozen Fruits and Vegetables - many types of organic fruits, vegetables, and fruit juices

Cascadian Farms
719 Metcalf
Sedro Wolley, WA 98284
(360) 855-0100
www.cfarm.com

ALL-FRUIT JAMS, SPREADS, AND SAUCES

Knudsen's all natural or organic fancy fruit spreads: most contain the specified fruit, white grape juice concentrate and fruit pectin. The apple butter contains apples and apple juice concentrate.

Knudsen and Sons, Inc.
Speedway Avenue
Chico, CA 95926
(530) 899-5000
www.knudsenjuices.com

Fiordifrutta Organic Fruit Spread: Organic raspberries (or the fruit for the variety of spread), organic apple juice, citrus pectin, citric acid.

Imported by Fiordifrutta Inc.
353 Christian Street
Oxford, CT 06478
Phone: (203) 267-3280

Wax Orchards Only Fruit Syrup: Puree of one fruit (raspberry, strawberry, blueberry, or marionberry) plus concentrate(s) of pineapple, pear, apple, peach, grape and/or lemon juice.
Wax Orchards Fudge Classic Topping: Unsweetened pineapple syrup, pear juice concentrate, Dutch cocoa, natural flavor.

Wax Orchards, Inc.
P.O. Box 25448
Seattle, WA 98665
(800) 634-6132
www.waxorchards.com

SOUPS AND BROTHS

Read soup labels carefully. Many soups contain wheat or wheat starch, modified food starch, sugar, yeast, MSG, etc. A few of the better soups are listed here.

Imagine Organic Free Range Chicken Broth: organic chicken broth (filtered water, organic chicken), organic onions, organic celery, organic carrots, sea salt, natural chicken flavor (no MSG or HVP), organic spices, organic expeller-pressed oil (canola and/or safflower and/or sunflower)

Imagine Foods
The Hain Celestial Group, Inc.
4600 Sleepytime Drive
Boulder, CO 80301
(800) 434-4246
www.hain-celestial.com

Shelton's All-Natural Chicken Broth, salt-free: chicken broth, onion, celery, spices. (The salted variety also contains chicken fat and sea salt)

Shelton's Premium Poultry
204 N. Loranne Avenue
Pomona, CA 91767
(800) 541-1833 or (909) 623-4361
www.sheltons.com

Hain Pure Foods "Healthy Naturals" Soups:
Chicken Broth: chicken broth, chicken fat, carrots, sea salt, onion powder, spices
Vegetarian Split Pea Soup: water, split peas, carrots, green peas, celery, onion powder, spices
Vegetarian Lentil Soup: water, lentils, celery, tomato paste, potato flour, onions, olive oil, garlic, spices
Black Bean Soup: water, black beans, tomato paste, celery, onions, sea salt, garlic, spices

The Hain Celestial Group, Inc.
4600 Sleepytime Drive
Boulder, CO 80301
(800) 434-4246
www.hain-celestial.com

Health Valley Natural Broths:
Chicken Broth: Filtered water, concentrated chicken broth, sea salt, onion powder, turmeric, ground celery seed, white pepper.
Beef Broth: Filtered water, beef extract, sea salt, onion powder, white pepper, ground celery seed.
Vegetable Broth: Filtered water, vegetable concentrates (carrot, onion, cabbage, shallot), honey, sea salt, onion powder, white pepper and celery seed.

Health Valley Foods
The Hain Celestial Group, Inc.
4600 Sleepytime Drive
Boulder, CO 80301
(800) 434-4246
www.healthvalley.com

Pacific Natural Foods broths: Several varieties, ingredients are given for two:
Pacific Organic Free Range Chicken Broth: Organic chicken broth (filtered water, organic chicken), organic chicken flavor (organic chicken, sea salt), sea salt, organic cane sweetener, onion powder, turmeric, natural flavor
Pacific Organic Vegetable Broth: Filtered water, organic carrots, organic tomato, organic celery, organic onions, organic garlic, organic leeks, sea salt, organic bay leaves, organic parsley, organic thyme.

Pacific Natural Foods, Inc.
19480 SW 97th Avenue
Tualatin, OR 97062
(503) 692-9666
www.pacificfoods.com

ALTERNATIVE MILK PRODUCTS

BUTTER

Mt. Sterling Cheese Corp. Pure Goat Milk Butter: goat cream only

Mt. Sterling Cheese Corporation
P.O. Box 103
Mt. Sterling, WI 54645
(608) 734-3151
http://grantcounty.org/visitor/farm.html

CHEESE

Soy, rice, almond, and hemp cheeses usually contain casein from cow's milk.

Goat Cheese

Mt. Sterling Cheese's Cheddar, Jack, etc.: pasteurized goat milk, salt, culture, and microbial enzymes

Mt. Sterling Cheese Corporation
P.O. Box 103
Mt. Sterling, WI 54645
(608) 734-3151
http://grantcounty.org/visitor/farm.html

MILK

Read the labels carefully because rice milk often contains legumes and soy milk often contains grains.

Goat milk

Meyenberg Goat Milk - available canned, powdered, ultrapasteurized and aseptic packed

Meyenberg Goat Milk
Jackson-Mitchell
P.O. Box 934
Turlock, CA 95381
(800) 891-GOAT
www.meyenberg.com

Nut milks such as almond and hazelnut:

Blue Diamond Unsweetened Vanilla Almond Breeze: Purified water, almonds, tapioca starch, natural vanilla flavor, other natural flavors, calcium carbonate, sea salt, potassium citrate, carageenan, soy lecithin, vitamin A palmitate, vitamin D2, and d-alpha tocopherol (natural vitamin E)

Blue Diamond Growers
1802 C Street
P.O. Box 1768
Sacramento CA, 95811
(916) 442-0771
www.bluediamond.com

Pacific Foods Hazelnut Non-Dairy Beverage: Filtered water, hazelnuts, brown rice sweetener, tri-calcium phosphate, sea salt, guar gum, xanthum gum, carageenan, carob bean gum, riboflavin (vitamin B2), vitamin A palmitate, vitamin D2.

Pacific Natural Foods, Inc.
19480 SW 97th Avenue
Tualatin, OR 97062
(503) 692-9666
www.pacificfoods.com

Oat milk

Pacific Foods Organic Oat Non-Dairy Drink, plain flavor: filtered water, organic oat groats, oat bran, tricalcium phosphate, sea salt, guar gum, xanthum gum, carrageenan, carob bean gum, riboflavin (B2), vitamin A palmitate, vitamin D2

Pacific Natural Foods, Inc.
19480 SW 97th Avenue
Tualatin, OR 97062
(503) 692-9666
www.pacificfoods.com

Rice milk

Rice Dream Rice Milk: filtered water, brown rice, safflower oil, vanilla, sea salt

Imagine Foods, Inc.
350 Cambridge Avenue, Suite 350
Palo Alto, CA 94306
(415) 327-1444
www.imaginefoods.com

Pacific Rice Non-Dairy Drink: water, brown rice, tricalcium phosphate, *L. acidophilus, L. bifidus,* guar gum, xanthum gum, carageenan, sea salt, vitamins A and D

Pacific Natural Foods, Inc.
19480 S.W. 97th Avenue
Tualatin, OR 97062
(503) 692-9666
www.pacificfoods.com

Soy milk

Edensoy Soy Milk (NOT gluten-free): Purified water, organic soybeans, malted cereal extract, Job's tears, barley, kombu, sea salt

Eden Foods, Inc.
701 Tecumseh Road
Clinton, MI 49236
(888) 424-EDEN (3336) or (517) 456-7424
www.edenfoods.com

Westsoy Soy Milk: filtered water, organic soybeans, brown rice syrup (possibly NOT gluten-free), vanilla, carageenan, sea salt

Westbrae Natural Foods
The Hain Celestial Group, Inc.
4600 Sleepytime Drive
Boulder, CO 80301
(800) 434-4246
www.westbrae.com

YOGURT:

Hollow Road Farms Sheep's Milk Yogurt: pasteurized sheep's milk, *L. bulgaricus, S. thermophilus, L. acidophilus, L. bifidus*

Hollow Road Farms
Old Chatham Sheepherding Company
155 Shaker Museum Road
Old Chatham, NY 12136
(888) SHEEP60 or (518) 794-7333
www.blacksheepcheese.com

Redwood Hill Farm Goat Milk Yogurt: pasteurized whole goat milk, tapioca, and living cultures *(L. bulgaricus, S. thermophilus, L. acidophilus, L. bifidus)*

Redwood Hill Farm
2064 Highway 116 North, Building 1
Sebastopol, CA 95472
(707) 823-8250
www.redwoodhill.com

White Wave Soy Yogurt: Filtered water, whole organic soybeans, organic evaporated cane juice, fruit (strawberries, cherries, blueberries, peaches, etc.), rice starch, dextrose (possibly from corn), natural flavors, tricalcium phosphate, pectin, citric acid, locust bean gum, annatto and turmeric (for color), yogurt cultures *(L. bulgaricus, S. thermophilus, L. acidophilus, B. bifidum, L. casei, L. rhamnosus)*.

White Wave Soy Foods, Inc.
1990 N. 57th Court
Boulder, CO 80301
(303) 443-3470
www.whitewave.com

BEVERAGES

COFFEE, INSTANT:

Mount Hagen Organic Instant Coffee is freeze-dried, available regular or decaffeinated, and sold in jars or single-serve packages.

Mount Hagen Organic Instant Coffee

Cafix of North America, Inc.
15 Prospect Street
Paramus NJ 07652
(201) 909-0808

Online source for Mount Hagen Coffee:

InterNatural Foods, LLC
300 Broadacres Drive
Bloomfield, New Jersey 07003
(973) 338-1499
www.internaturalfoods.com/MountHagen/MountHagen.html

ALL-FRUIT SODA:

Knudsen Fruit Spritzers

Knudsen and Sons, Inc.
Speedway Avenue
Chico, CA 95926
(530) 899-5000
www.knudsenjuices.com

WINE, GLUTEN-FREE ORGANIC:

Bonterra Organic Wines
Bonterra Vineyards
2231 McNab Ranch Road
Ukiah, CA 95482
www.bonterra.com

Sources of Special Ingredients, Products and Services

This section lists sources of special ingredients needed for cooking, products, and services that may not always be easy to find locally. Also see pages 187 to 208 for sources of commercially prepared foods. Most of these companies sell products and services in addition to those listed below. Visit their websites for up-to-date information about all of their products and services.

DISINFECTANTS

Nutribiotic™ for disinfecting produce
N.E.E.D.S
6666 Manlius Center Road
East Syracuse, NY 13057
(800) 634-1380
www.needs.com

E.G.G. (Ethylene Gas Guardian)

WayChem, Inc.
P.O. Box 1450
84 Allegiance Circle
Evanston, WY, 82931
(307) 444-2000
www.4theegg.com

FLOURS, GRAINS, and GRAIN ALTERNATIVES

Amaranth grain, flour and cereal

Nu-World Amaranth, Inc.
P. O. Box 2202
Naperville, IL 60540
(630) 369-6819
www.nuworldfoods.com

Arrowroot

Authentic Foods
1850 W. 168th Street, Suite B
Gardena, CA 90247
(800) 806-4737 or (310) 366-7612
www.authenticfoods.com

Buckwheat flour

Arrowhead Mills
The Hain Celestial Group, Inc.
4600 Sleepytime Drive
Boulder, CO 80301
(800) 434-4246
www.hain-celestial.com

Cassava meal (also called manioc flour)

Sundial Herbal Products
3609 Boston Post Road
Bronx, NY 10466
(718) 798-3962
www.sundialherbs.com/html /other_products.html

Chestnut flour

Gold Mine Natural Food Company
7805 Arjons Drive
San Diego, CA 92126
(800) 475-FOOD
www.goldminenaturalfood.com

Kamut flour

Arrowhead Mills
The Hain Celestial Group, Inc.
4600 Sleepytime Drive
Boulder, CO 80301
(800) 434-4246
www.hain-celestial.com

Millet grain and flour

Bob's Red Mill Natural Foods Inc.
5209 S.E. International Way
Milwaukie, OR 97222
(800) 349-2173 or (503) 654-3215
www.bobsredmill.com

Quinoa grain, flour and pasta

The Quinoa Corporation
P.O. Box 279
Gardena, CA. 90248
(310) 217-8125
www.quinoa.net

Rice flour – brown, white, or sweet rice

Authentic Foods
1850 W. 168th Street, Suite B
Gardena, CA 90247
(800) 806-4737 or (310) 366-7612
www.authenticfoods.com

Rye flour

Arrowhead Mills
The Hain Celestial Group, Inc.
4600 Sleepytime Drive
Boulder, CO 80301
(800) 434-4246
www.hain-celestial.com

Sorghum (milo) flour

Authentic Foods
1850 W. 168th Street, Suite B
Gardena, CA 90247
(800) 806-4737 or (310) 366-7612
www.authenticfoods.com

Spelt grain, flour, and pasta

Purity Foods, Inc.
2871 W. Jolly Road
Okemos, MI 48864
(517) 351-9231
www.purityfoods.com

Tapioca flour

Authentic Foods
1850 W. 168th Street, Suite B
Gardena, CA 90247
(800) 806-4737 or (310) 366-7612
www.authenticfoods.com

Teff grain and flour

Bob's Red Mill
Natural Foods Inc.
5209 S.E. International Way
Milwaukie, OR 97222
(800) 349-2173 or (503) 654-3215
www.bobsredmill.com

INGREDIENTS FOR BAKING, MISCELLANEOUS

Baking powder, corn-free

Featherweight Baking Powder
The Hain Celestial Group, Inc.
4600 Sleepytime Drive
Boulder, CO 80301
(800) 434-4246
www.hain-celestial.com

Chocolate chips, dairy, soy and gluten-free

Enjoy Life™ Semi-Sweet Chocolate Chips
Enjoy Life™ Natural Brands, LLC
3810 N. River Road
Schiller Park, IL 60176
(888-503-6569 (888-50-ENJOY)
www.enjoylifenb.com

Flavorings, natural, gluten-, corn- and alcohol-free

The Spicery Shoppe Natural Flavorings
The Spicery Shoppe
1525 Brook Drive
Downers Grove, IL 60515
(800) 323-1301 or (630) 932-8100

Frontier Natural Flavorings*

Frontier Natural Products Co-op
P.O. Box 299
3021 78th Street
Norway, IA 52318
(800) 669-3275
www.frontierherb.com

*Note: Some Frontier flavorings such as vanilla are corn-, alcohol-, and gluten-free; others are not.

Gum, Guar and Xanthum

Authentic Foods
1850 W. 168th Street, Suite B
Gardena, CA 90247
(800) 806-4737 or (310) 366-7612
www.authenticfoods.com

Oils and non-hydrogenated, trans-fat free shortening

Spectrum Naturals™ Oils
Spectrum Naturals™ Organic All
Vegetable Shortening: Palm oil only (soy-free)
Spectrum Organic Products, Inc.
5341 Old Redwood Highway, Suite 400
Petaluma, CA 94954
www.spectrumorganics.com

Rye flavor powder (gluten-free)

Authentic Foods
1850 W. 168th Street, Suite B
Gardena, CA 90247
(800) 806-4737 or (310) 366-7612
www.authenticfoods.com

Unbuffered vitamin C powder, cassava source, made by Allergy Research Group, for baking and salads

Professional Supplement Center
2427 Porter Lake Drive
Sarasota, FL 34230
(888) 245-5000
www.professionalsupplementcenter.com

Yeast, active dry and quick-rise, gluten-, corn- and preservative-free

Red Star Yeast and SAF Yeast
Universal Foods Corporation
Consumer Service Center
433 E. Michigan Street
Milwaukee, WI 53202
(414) 271-6755
www.redstaryeast.com

The Red Star Yeast company is a great information source but does not sell direct to consumers. To purchase Red Star™ or SAF™ yeast in 1 or 2-pound bags, contact:

King Arthur Flour Baker's Catalogue
P.O. Box 876
Norwich, Vermont 05055
(800) 827-6836
www.kingarthurflour.com

KITCHEN EQUIPMENT

Apple peeler/corer, crank-style

Progressive International Corp.
6111 S. 228th Street
Kent, WA 98032
(800) 426-7101 or (253) 850-6111
www.progressiveintl.com
Also sold on **Amazon.com.**

Bread machines, measuring cups, etc.

King Arthur Flour Baker's Catalogue
P.O. Box 876
Norwich, Vermont 05055
(800) 827-6836
www.kingarthurflour.com

Coffee systems, French drip requiring a paper filter

Melitta USA Inc.
13925 58th Street North
Clearwater, Florida 33760
(888) 635-4882 (888-MELITTA)
www.melitta.com

To see any Melitta French drip system online go to:
http://shop.melitta.com/search. asp?SKW=MACM

For the Ready-Set-Joe Travel Mug and Cone system ($8.99 at the time of this writing) go to:
http://shop.melitta.com/itemdy00. asp?T1=64+081&Cat=

Coffee systems, French drip with a gold mesh filter (Item # 53-300, $12.95 at the time of this writing)

Lehman's
One Lehman's Circle
P.O. Box 270
Kidron, OH 44636
(888) 438-5346
www.lehmans.com

Lettuce keeper

Harriet Carter Gifts, Inc.
425 Stump Road
North Wales, PA 19455
(800)-377-7878
www.harrietcarter.com

The lettuce keeper costs $7.98 at the time of this writing.

NUT PRODUCTS

Almond flour/meal

Authentic Foods
1850 W. 168th Street, Suite B
Gardena, CA 90247
(800) 806-4737 or (310) 366-7612
www.authenticfoods.com

Coconut, finely shredded unsweetened

Jerry's Nut House, Inc.
2101 Humboldt Street
Denver, CO 80205
(303) 861-2262

Pecan meal

King Arthur Flour Baker's Catalogue
P.O. Box 876
Norwich, VT 05055
(800) 827-6836
www.kingarthurflour.com

PROFESSIONALS, HEALTH

Physicians who specialize in the diagnosis and treatment of food allergies

American Academy of Environmental Medicine
7701 East Kellogg, Suite 625
Wichita, KS 67207
(316) 684-5500
www.aaem.com

American College for Advancement in Medicine
23121 Verdugo Drive, Suite 204
Laguna Hills, CA 92653
(888) 439-6891, (800) 532-3688 or
(949) 583-7666
www.acam.org

Nutritionists

International & American Associations of Clinical Nutritionists
15280 Addison Road, Suite 130
Addison, TX 75001
(972) 407-9089
www.iaacn.org

SPICES

Chile pequin

Fernandez Chile Company
8267 County Road 10 South
Alamosa, CO 81101
(719) 589-6043

SWEETENERS

Agave

Madhava agave nectar, light and amber
Madhava Honey
4689 Ute Highway
Lyons, CO 80540
(303) 823-5166
www.madhavahoney.com/agave.htm

Date sugar

NOW Natural Foods *(order through your health food store)*
395 S. Glen Ellyn Road
Bloomingdale, IL 60108
(800) 283-3500
www.nowfoods.com

Fruit Sweet™, Grape Sweet™, and Pear Sweet™

Wax Orchards, Inc.
P.O. Box 25448
Seattle, WA 98665
(800) 634-6132
www.waxorchards.com

THICKENERS

ThickenUp™
Novartis Pharmaceuticals
One Health Plaza
East Hanover, NJ 07936-1080
Phone: 862-778-8300
FAX: 973-781-8265
www.pharma.us.novartis.com

Safe Food Handling Practices

The principles of food safety are simple. Just don't give bacteria, viruses, and parasites what they need to live and grow, and kill them by exposure them to plenty of what they cannot tolerate.

Temperature

Bacteria like a nice warm environment. Lukewarm food is an ideal growth substrate for them, but your food will be safe as long as it is very cold or very hot. The temperature in your refrigerator should be 41°F or less. Check it with a thermometer occasionally and adjust the temperature control dial until it maintains a temperature of about 40°F. At this temperature, bacteria will not be killed but neither will they multiply rapidly. Keep all animal foods and most plant foods, with the exception of ripening fruit, in the refrigerator or freezer at all times. Freezer temperatures will kill some parasites and bacteria.

Food safety should be your first priority after grocery shopping. Put all of your groceries away promptly when you get home giving meat, poultry, fish, dairy products, and other refrigerated and frozen foods the highest priority. Freeze meat, poultry and fish if you are not planning to eat them within one or two days after purchase.

Don't let leftovers sit at room temperature after dinner. Refrigerate or freeze them promptly and always within two hours of when they were prepared.

When refrigerators were new, people were advised to let hot foods cool to room temperature before putting them into the refrigerator. It is true that this saves your refrigerator work, but leaving food out on the counter to cool for an extended time period is not a safe practice from the standpoint of bacteria. The safest and most efficient way to handle hot leftovers is to divide them into small portions for storage, which allows the heat to dissipate more quickly, and to set them on a rack to cool briefly (not all the way to room temperature) before putting them into the refrigerator.

Cook foods thoroughly. Dr. Leo Galland recommends cooking all animal foods conventionally because microwave ovens often have hot spots and cold spots, and certain areas of the food may not reach a high enough temperature to kill bacteria and parasites which may be present.[1] When you cook vegetables in a microwave, stir them during the cooking process to insure sufficient heating of all parts of the food.

For conventional cooking of large cuts of meat and poultry, use a meat ther-mometer to determine when they are done. Turkeys should be cooked until the temperature in the deepest part of the breast and thigh is 180° to185°F. Do not let the thermometer touch bone. Beef roasts can be cooked to a range of thermometer temperatures depending on how well done you like your meat. Beef roasts and steaks are safe when cooked rare because they are cuts of muscle meat that are sterile on the inside. Only the cut surfaces will be contaminated with bacteria. Therefore, the entire inside of the roast does not need to reach a temperature high enough to kill bacteria. Ground meat, however, is another story. It is basically all cut surfaces which are subject to bacterial contamination. Therefore, cook your ground meat until the pink is completely gone. Pork should always be cooked thoroughly to kill the parasite *Trichenella spiralis.* Test pork roasts with a meat thermometer and leave them in the oven until the temperature registers at least 170°F in the deepest part of the meat.

Frozen meat or poultry should be thawed in the refrigerator rather than by allowing it to stand at room temperature. If you can't wait as longs as it will take to thaw your turkey in the refrigerator (and in the case of a large bird, it may be several days), you can thaw it in a sink of cool water. Check the bird and replace the water with fresh cool water regularly. When the turkey feels spongy, remove it from the water and refrigerate or cook it immediately. Small cuts of meat may be defrosted in your microwave oven but only if you are going to cook them immedi-ately after thawing them this way because they may develop hot spots.

Fish is highly perishable and should be kept cold from the minute it is taken from the water until it is cooked. Never buy fish from a fisherman's truck; only buy from reputable markets which get their fish from government-inspected fisheries. After you purchase fresh fish, get it home and into the refrigerator quickly. Cook fresh fish within one or at most two days of purchase. Keep frozen fish frozen until you plan to eat it; then thaw it in the refrigerator. If it is not thawed in time for dinner, you can cook fish starting from frozen although it will take a few minutes longer to be done. Always cook fish thoroughly. Test it for doneness by piercing it with a fork. If it flakes easily and is opaque throughout, it has been cooked enough. If you poach fish, it is impossible to dry it out and you can err on the side of over-cooking it without consequence.

Eggs should be cooked until both the white and yolk are set. Cook scrambled eggs until there is no liquid egg remaining. If you like your eggs soft-cooked or prefer fried eggs with soft yolks, use pasteurized eggs. Get eggs into the refrigerator as soon as you get them home from the store. If there happens to be a contami-nated egg in your carton and you leave it at room temperature, the bacteria will multiply to a number that is much more likely to make you sick if the eggs are undercooked.

Chemical environment

Bacteria, parasites, and viruses are affected by the chemical environment in which they find themselves as well as by temperature. We can exploit the sensitivity of harmful organisms to chemicals to make our food safe.

When you plan to eat fresh fruits or vegetables raw, for maximum safety you should disinfect them as well as washing them. *In Guess What Came to Dinner*, Ann Louise Gittleman suggests that raw fruits and vegetables be disinfected by soaking them in a solution of ½ teaspoon of Clorox™ for each gallon of water. Thin skinned fruits and leafy vegetables should be soaked for 15 minutes and thick skinned produce should be soaked for 30 minutes.[2] Dr. Leo Galland recommends soaking fruits and vegetables in a solution of 2 teaspoons of 3% hydrogen peroxide to each gallon of water.[3] Nutribiotic™, a grapefruit seed extract, can also be used for disinfecting foods. In laboratory testing, this non-toxic food-based extract has been shown to be effective against a wide range of bacteria, yeast, fungi, and parasites. At our house, as soon as we get home from the grocery store, any produce we plan to eat raw is soaked for 30 minutes in a sink full of cool water with about 30 drops of Nutribiotic™ added. If you purchase fragile produce, such as berries, you may wish to hold off on soaking them until right before you plan to eat them. Nutribiotic™ can be purchased at most health food stores, or for a mail-order source, see page 209.

A few simple practices will keep bacteria and other organisms from spreading in your home. Dr. Leo Galland says hand washing is a very effective way to remove pathogens and prevent the transmission of disease of all kinds.[4] As soon as you come home, wash your hands to keep from bringing bacteria, viruses, or parasites into your own environment. Before you begin cooking, every time you cook, wash your hands thoroughly with warm water and soap, sudsing for a few minutes. If you handle raw meat or poultry while cooking, wash your hands thoroughly again. Any time you think you may have touched something that could possibly be contaminated while cooking, re-wash your hands.

Cutting boards can also spread infection. Do not use wooden cutting boards because they can harbor bacteria in grooves or cracks in the wood and are nearly impossible to clean thoroughly. Glass or plastic cutting boards can be washed in soap and hot water or put in the dishwasher to clean and disinfect them. If you use a cutting board for raw meat, poultry, or fish, wash it thoroughly before using it for anything else. Food poisoning bacteria can be easily transmitted by cutting raw meat on a cutting board and then using the same cutting board to cut vegetables that will be eaten raw.

Your kitchen counters should be kept thoroughly clean and disinfected regularly. Wash your counters with hot soapy water and/or with a disinfectant on a regular or daily basis. Also wash and disinfect them whenever they are dirty or especially when they may have become contaminated with juices from raw meat or poultry. I like to disinfect our kitchen counters routinely every day as I am cleaning up the kitchen after dinner. For maximum safety, first wash your counters with hot soapy water to remove food and grease. (Disinfectants will only work if they can get to the germs, and grease and dirt protect them from chemicals). Then disinfect the counters by moistening a piece of paper towel with hot water and a teaspoon of Clorox™ or a good squirt of Nutribiotic™ and wiping the counters down with the disinfectant-soaked paper towel.

Be careful of how you wash dishes. Do not leave your dishes soaking for a prolonged time because the dishwater will cool to a lukewarm temperature where bacteria thrive. The food that is left on the dishes will dissolve in the water, making a nice soup for bacteria to enjoy. Keep your dishwater hot and soapy. If you must leave the dishes half-done and the water cools, replace it with hot soapy water before you finish washing your dishes. Whether you wash the dishes by hand or in a dishwasher, it is most hygienic let them air dry so you don't add bacteria to them with your hands or a dish towel.

Dishwashers which have the water temperature set high enough are excellent for killing bacteria. However, the hot water and detergent must be able to get to the bacteria. If you put your dishes into the dishwasher with dried food on them that doesn't come off in washing, bacteria can be lurking under that food. Clean visible food off before loading dishes into the dishwasher.

Throw away your dishrags and sponges. This is one area where health issues should take precedence over environment concerns. Dr. Leo Galland recommends that we use paper towels to wipe counters and other kitchen surfaces, not a sponge or dishrag. For washing dishes, use disposable dishrags such as HandiWipes™ and replace them often rather than using a sponge or cloth dishrag. Because bacteria love to grow in wet sponges and dishrags, the kitchen sponge is usually the most unsanitary object in the home.

If you follow these practices routinely, you kitchen will never be a source of food borne illness.

Footnotes

1. Galland, Leo, M.D., *The Four Pillars of Healing*, Random House, New York, 1997, p. 215.
2. Gittleman, Ann Louise, *Guess What Came to Dinner: Parasites and Your Health*, Avery Publishing Group, Inc., Garden Park, NY, 1993, p. 128.
3. Galland, p. 215.
4. Galland, p. 214.

The Spelt-Wheat Debate

If you have celiac disease, an allergy to gluten itself, or gluten intolerance of any kind, you should eat neither spelt nor wheat because both contain gluten. The information in this section is of no personal value to you, so skip ahead if you wish. However, if you are allergic to wheat but do not have gluten intolerance, you may – or may not – be able to eat spelt. Have your doctor test you for it and advise you based on the test results.

When shopping for spelt products, be aware that a great deal of confusion has risen concerning spelt recently. The United States Government now requires that foods be labeled to indicate whether the food contains any of eight food allergens. As part of the implementation of this law, the FDA has declared that spelt is wheat. Although spelt and wheat are indeed closely related, they are two different species in the same genus. Spelt is *Triticum spelta* and wheat is *Triticum aestivum*. When asked why they had decided that spelt is wheat, an FDA official said that it was because spelt contains gluten. (They had no answer to the question of whether rye would also be considered wheat because it contains gluten, and indeed, bags of rye flour in the health food store are still labeled "wheat-free"). Spelt does indeed contain gluten and should not be eaten by anyone who is gluten-sensitive or has celiac disease, but the presence of gluten does not make spelt wheat. However, under the new law, packages of spelt products must be labeled "Contains wheat."

There are a variety of reasons for the tolerance some wheat-allergic patients have for spelt. All grains contain components in addition to gluten to which a person may develop an allergy. If you are allergic to one of them, but not gluten, you may tolerate spelt.

There are other differences between wheat and spelt. The gluten in spelt behaves differently than the gluten in wheat in cooking. It is extremely difficult to make seitan from spelt. (Seitan is a meat substitute that is almost pure gluten). When making it from wheat, a process of soaking in hot water is used to remove the starch from the gluten protein. If the same process is followed with spelt, the protein structure also dissolves in the hot water. Spelt seitan must be washed by hand very carefully under running cold water.

Because the gluten in spelt is more soluble than wheat gluten, making yeast bread with spelt is also different than making it with wheat. The individual gluten molecules join up more readily to form long chains and sheets that trap the gas produced by yeast. This means that it is possible to over-knead spelt bread. There are some bread machines that work quite well for wheat and even other allergy breads but are unacceptable for spelt bread because they knead so vigorously that they over-develop the gluten. See pages 41 to 42 of this book and pages 32 to 33 of *Easy Breadmaking for Special Diets* (described on the last pages of this book) for recommendations about bread machines to use for making spelt bread.

It is possible that the greater solubility of spelt protein makes it easier to digest than wheat. Undoubtedly, most people have had much less prior exposure to spelt than to wheat resulting in less opportunity to become allergic to spelt. Whatever the reason, there are many people who suffer allergic reactions after eating wheat but do not react to spelt. (I have talked to hundreds of them). Restricting one's diet unnecessarily, as the confusion generated by new labeling law will undoubtedly lead people to do, is counterproductive to good nutrition. Consult your doctor about your own food allergy test results and follow the diet recommended for you, but do not unnecessarily restrict spelt consumption based on the faulty logic behind the new government labeling requirements.

References
Helpful Books and Websites

BOOKS

Crook, William G. M.D., *Detecting Your Hidden Allergies*, Professional Books, Inc., Box 3246, Jackson, TN 38303, 1988.

Crook, William G., M.D., *The Yeast Connection*. Professional Books, Jackson, Tennessee, 38303, 1983. (Dr. Crook wrote a series of "Yeast Connection" books such as *The Yeast Connection and the Woman* which are all very useful).

Crook, William G., M.D. and Marjorie Hurt Jones, R.N. *The Yeast Connection Cookbook*. Professional Books, Jackson, Tennessee, 38303, 1989.

Dumke, Nicolette M. *Allergy Cooking With Ease*. Starburst Publishers, Lancaster, PA, 1992; Allergy Adapt, Inc., 1877 Polk Avenue, Louisville, CO 80027, Revised edition, 2007.

Dumke, Nicolette M. *Easy Breadmaking for Special Diets*. Allergy Adapt, Inc., 1877 Polk Avenue, Louisville, CO 80027, 1995; Revised edition, 2007.

Dumke, Nicolette M. *Easy Cooking for Special Diets: How to Cook for Weight Loss/ Blood Sugar Control, Food Allergy, Heart Healthy, Diabetic and "Just Healthy" Diets – Even if You've Never Cooked Before*. Allergy Adapt, Inc., 1877 Polk Avenue, Louisville, CO 80027, 2007.

Dumke, Nicolette M. *Gluten-Free Without Rice*. Allergy Adapt, Inc., 1877 Polk Avenue, Louisville, CO 80027, 2007.

Dumke, Nicolette M. *The Low Dose Immunotherapy Handbook: Recipes and Lifestyle Advice for Patients on LDA and EPD Treatment*. Allergy Adapt, Inc., 1877 Polk Avenue, Louisville, CO 80027, 2003.

Dumke, Nicolette M. *The Ultimate Food Allergy Cookbook and Survival Guide*. Allergy Adapt, Inc., 1877 Polk Avenue, Louisville, CO 80027, 2007.

Galland, Leo, M.D. *The Four Pillars of Healing.* Random House, New York, NY, 1997.

Hagman, Bette. *The Gluten-Free Gourmet: Living Well Without Wheat.* Henry Holt and Company, New York, NY, 1990. Revised edition, 2000.

Jones, Marjorie Hurt, R.N. *The Allergy Self-Help Cookbook.* Rodale Press, Emmaus, Pennsylvania, 1984, Revised edition, 2001.

Lewis, Sondra K. with Lonette Dietrich Blakely. *Allergy and Candida Cooking: Understanding and Implementing Plans for Healing.* Canary Connect Publications, 605 Holiday Road, Coralville, IA 52241-1016, 2006.

Randolph, Theron G., M.D. and Ralph W. Moss, Ph.D. *An Alternative Approach to Allergies.* Bantam Books, New York, 1980.

Zolezzi, Anthony, Linda Bonvie and Bill Bonvie. *Chemical-Free Kids: The Organic Sequel.* ASM Books, La Habra, CA, 2008.

WEBSITES

Help for Celiacs:
Gluten Intolerance Group of North America – www.gluten.net
   This website includes a restaurant database at www.glutenfreerestaurants.org/find.php. See page 22 for more about this service.
Celiac.com – www.celiac.com

Help for those with food allergies:
Food Allergy.org – www.food-allergy.org
Optimal Health Resource Laboratories – www.yorkallergyusa.com
   (for allergy testing)

Information about LDA and EPD:
Low Dose Immunotherapy page – www.food-allergy.org/epd.html
Dr. Shrader's EPD and LDA page – www.drshrader.com/news.htm

Products that can be used on celiac and food allergy diets:
See pages 187 to 214 for websites of companies that produce and sell special diet foods and products.

Table of Measurements

You may occasionally need to measure less-common amounts of ingredients such as ⅜ cup or ⅛ teaspoon. The easiest and most accurate way to do this is to have a liquid measuring cup with ⅛ cup markings, a set of dry measuring cups that contains a ⅛ cup measure, and a set of measuring spoons that has a ⅛ teaspoon. Such kitchen equipment is available from the King Arthur Flour Baker's Catalogue (See "Sources," page 212). But while you are waiting for your measuring cups and spoons to arrive or if you need to halve, double, or triple recipes, use this table.

⅛ teaspoon	= ½ of your ¼ teaspoon measure	
⅜ teaspoon	= ¼ teaspoon + ⅛ teaspoon	
⅝ teaspoon	= ½ teaspoon + ⅛ teaspoon	
¾ teaspoon	= ½ teaspoon + ¼ teaspoon	
⅞ teaspoon	= ½ teaspoon + ¼ teaspoon + ⅛ teaspoon	
1 teaspoon	= ⅓ tablespoon	= ⅙ fluid ounce
1½ teaspoons	= ½ tablespoon	= ¼ fluid ounce
3 teaspoons	= 1 tablespoon	= ½ fluid ounce
½ tablespoon	= 1½ teaspoons	= ¼ fluid ounce
1 tablespoon	= 3 teaspoons	= ½ fluid ounce
2 tablespoons*	= ⅛ cup	= 1 fluid ounce
4 tablespoons	= ¼ cup	= 2 fluid ounces
5⅓ tablespoons	= ⅓ cup	= 2⅔ fluid ounces
8 tablespoons	= ½ cup	= 4 fluid ounces
16 tablespoons	= 1 cup	= 8 fluid ounces
⅛ cup	= 2 tablespoons*	= 1 fluid ounce
¼ cup	= 4 tablespoons	= 2 fluid ounces
⅜ cup	= ¼ cup + 2 tablespoons*	= 3 fluid ounces
⅝ cup	= ½ cup + 2 tablespoons*	= 5 fluid ounces
¾ cup	= ½ cup + ¼ cup	= 6 fluid ounces
⅞ cup	= ¾ cup + 2 tablespoons*	= 7 fluid ounces
	OR ½ cup + ¼ cup + 2 tablespoons*	
1 cup	= ½ pint	= 8 fluid ounces
1 pint	= 2 cups	= 16 fluid ounces
1 quart	= 4 cups OR 2 pints	= 32 fluid ounces
1 gallon	= 4 quarts	= 128 fluid ounces

*Note: In my experience, measuring tablespoons are all a little scanty of $\frac{1}{16}$ cup so 2 tablespoons is a little short of ⅛ cup. Therefore, if you need to measure, for example, ⅜ cup of liquid and do not have a measuring cup with ⅛ cup markings, it will probably be more accurate to eyeball an amount halfway between ¼ cup and ½ cup than to use ¼ cup plus two tablespoons.

Index to Recipes by Grain Use

To help those on a rotation diet find recipes made with the grain they need for each diet day, this index lists the recipes in this book according to the major grain or grain alternative that they contain. The recipes that do not contain a grain or grain alternative, such as those for main dishes, vegetables, etc., are not listed in this index but can be found by name in the "General Index," page 226. Arrowroot and tapioca are used as binders or thickeners in many recipes in this book; since they are not the main flour-type ingredient in any recipes, they are not included in the listing below.

General Index

Recipes appear in *italics*. Informational sections appear in standard type.

W

X

Y

Z

Books to Help You with
Your Special Diet

In these times of economic downturn, what is a person on a special diet to do? *Allergy and Celiac Diets With Ease: Money and Time Saving Solutions for Food Allergy and Celiac Diets* provides solutions to both the economic and time challenges you face on your diet. It shows how to shop economically, cook without spending all day in the kitchen, stock your kitchen for efficiency and good health, make the best use of your appliances, have good times with friends and family without breaking the bank, get organized, and be able to do this in limited time. This book contains over 160 money-saving, quick and easy recipes for allergy and celiac diets. Over 140 of them are gluten-free. It includes extensive reference sections including "Sources" and "Special Diet Resources" sections to help you find the foods you need. A list of helpful books and websites (even an online celiac/special diet restaurant search database) is also included.

ISBN 978-1-887624-17-6 . . . .$19.95

The Ultimate Food Allergy Cookbook and Survival Guide: How to Cook with Ease for Food Allergies and Recover Good Health gives you everything you need to survive and recover from food allergies. It contains medical information about the diagnosis of food allergies, health problems that can be caused by food allergies, and your options for treatment. The book includes a rotation diet that is free from common food allergens such as wheat, milk, eggs, corn, soy, yeast, beef, legumes, citrus fruits, potatoes, tomatoes, and more. Instructions are given on how to personalize the standard rotation diet to meet your individual needs and fit your food preferences. It contains 500 recipes that can be used with (or independently of) the diet. Extensive reference sections include a listing of commercially prepared foods for allergy diets and sources for special foods, services, and products.

ISBN 978-1-887624-08-4 . . . .$24.95

Gluten-Free Without Rice introduces you to gluten-free grains and grain alternatives other than rice such as teff, millet, sorghum, amaranth, quinoa, buckwheat, tapioca, arrowroot, corn, potato starch, and more. It gives you over 75 delicious recipes for muffins, crackers, bread, pancakes, waffles, granola, main and side dishes, cookies, and desserts. (Even ice cream cones!) With this book you can cook easily for a gluten-free diet without relying on rice. Whether you have celiac disease or food allergies, this book will make it easier and more enjoyable to stay on your diet and will help you to improve your health.

ISBN 978-1-887624-15-2 . . . .$9.95

Allergy Cooking With Ease (**Revised Edition**). This classic all-purpose allergy cookbook was out of print and now is making a comeback in a revised edition. It includes all the old favorite recipes of the first edition plus many new recipes and new foods. It contains over 300 recipes for baked goods, main dishes, soups, salads, vegetables, ethnic dishes, desserts, and more. Informational sections of the book are also totally updated, including the extensive "Sources" section.

ISBN 978-1-887624-10-7 . . . .$19.95

Easy Breadmaking for Special Diets contains over 200 recipes for allergy, heart healthy, low fat, low sodium, yeast-free, controlled carbohydrate, diabetic, celiac, and low calorie diets. It includes recipes for breads of all kinds, tortillas, bread and tortilla based main dishes, and desserts. Use your bread machine, food processor, mixer, or electric tortilla maker to make the bread YOU need quickly and easily.

Revised Edition – ISBN 978-1-887624-11-4 . . . . $19.95

Original Edition Bargain Book – ISBN 1-887624-02-3 . . . . **SALE!** - $9.95

   With the bargain book we will include an insert of updated pages about current bread machines and the tortilla recipes from the new edition.

Easy Cooking for Special Diets: How to Cook for Weight Loss/Blood Sugar Control, Food Allergy, Heart Healthy, Diabetic and "Just Healthy" Diets – Even if You've Never Cooked Before. This book contains everything you need to know to stay on your diet plus 265 recipes complete with nutritional analyses and diabetic exchanges. It also includes basics such as how to grocery shop, equip your kitchen, handle food safely, time management, information on nutrition, and sources of special foods.

ISBN 978-1-887624-09-1 . . . . $24.95

The Low Dose Immunotherapy Handbook: Recipes and Lifestyle Tips for Patients on LDA and EPD Treatment gives 80 recipes for patients on low dose immunotherapy treatment for their food allergies. It also includes organizational information to help you get ready for your shots.

ISBN: 978-1-887624-07-7 . . . .$9.95

How to Cope With Food Allergies When You're Short on Time is a booklet of time saving tips and recipes to help you stick to your allergy or gluten-free diet with the least amount of time and effort.

. . . . $4.95 or FREE with the order of two other books on these pages

Order these books on-line by going to
www.food-allergy.org,
by mail using the order form on the next page
or from Amazon.com at **www.amazon.com**.

Mail your order form and check to:
Allergy Adapt, Inc.
1877 Polk Avenue
Louisville, CO 80027

Questions? Call 303-666-8253
or email foodalle@food-allergy.org.

Shipping for mail-in orders:

IF YOU ARE ORDERING JUST ONE BOOK, FOR SHIPPING ADD:
$5.00 for any one of the starred (*) books above.
$2.00 for any one of the non-starred books above.

TO ORDER MORE THAN ONE BOOK, FOR SHIPPING ADD:
$6.50 for up to three starred* and up to two non-starred books
$9.00 for up to four starred* and up to two non-starred books
$11.00 for up to eight starred* and up to three non-starred books

Call 303-666-8253 for international shipping rates or if you have questions about shipping calculations or large quantity orders.

Thank you for your order!

Order Form

Send to:

Name: _____

Street address: _____

City, State, ZIP code: _____

Phone number (for questions about order): _____

Item	Quantity	Price	Total
Allergy and Celiac Diets With Ease*		$19.95	
The Ultimate Food Allergy Cookbook and Survival Guide*		$24.95	
Gluten-Free Without Rice		$9.95	
Allergy Cooking With Ease*		$19.95	

Easy Breadmaking for Special Diets* –
    Original Edition Bargain Book
    Revised Edition
		$9.95
		 $19.95	

Easy Cooking for Special Diets*		$24.95	
The Low Dose How Immunotherapy Handbook		$9.95	
How to Cope with Food Allergies When You're Short on Time		$4.95 or **FREE**	
Order any TWO of the first seven books above and get ***How to Cope*** **FREE!**	Subtotal		
	Shipping – See chart on page 237		
	Colorado residents add 4.1% sales tax		
	Total		

Printed in the United States
153165LV00003B/7/P